MEDICAL CARE FOR MOUNTAIN CLIMBERS

for
Tony Holmyard

MEDICAL CARE FOR MOUNTAIN CLIMBERS

Peter Steele

Line drawings by
Phoebe Bullock

William Heinemann Medical Books Ltd
London

First published 1976

ISBN 0 433 31560 1

Typeset in Great Britain
by Reproduction Drawings Ltd
and printed by Chapel River Press

Contents

Introduction

Dear Reader,

This book is written for you, the active mountain climber out on the hills. It aims to help you muster your wits in order to keep a casualty alive in those first few shattering minutes after an accident, and to prevent him worsening before he can reach skilled care. You may be a teacher taking a party of schoolchildren on Dartmoor or over Ben Alligin, a virtuoso on the north face of the Piz Badile or a young doctor in some wild valley beyond Dhaulagiri. Your medical knowledge will vary widely, therefore pitching the book at the right level is difficult. If it appears too facile at times, too complex at others, I ask your patience. I have tried to put myself in your boots throughout, because I know how frightening it is to have a serious accident on your hands without adequate experience or equipment to manage it.

I have avoided lists of symptoms and tasks to be learned by rote because if you understand the principles of the problem on hand you should be able to work out what action is appropriate. You may have limited medical knowledge, but using maximum common sense is what casualty care is all about. Care must be total. It means looking after the casualty as a whole person — frightened, in pain, anxious — not just splinting his broken leg. (Women readers please excuse my chauvinism in always referring to the victim as male, but this is an insurmountable technicality of grammar. I know who I would choose for staying power.)

Jargon bedevils my profession and is the cloak under which we doctors retain our mystique. While writing this book my old friend and mentor the Shorter Oxford English Dictionary lay ready at my left elbow; my medical encyclopaedia remained unopened on my study shelf. In the first draft of the book I tried to explain a technical situation in plain English, then I put the medical term in brackets as if to mollify my colleagues lest they think I am talking down to them. A friend, having read it, asked if I was trying to educate her. So I struck out most of the bracketed terms unless they were either common English parlance or made the meaning clearer.

In the text drugs are mentioned only by their approved names and without dosages; these may be found at the end of the book in the pharmacopoeia that includes only such drugs already mentioned. I have selected them on expert advice and I take any blame for omissions or controversial choices.

The drawings are a supplement for the written word, not a lazy man's way of skipping through the book. Each was carefully planned, then pruned and redrawn until it showed only such details as are meaningful in their context. My skilful artist and friend, Phoebe Bullock, remained ever patient and her contribution to the book is self-evident.

For a Jack-of-all-trades to write a book covering so wide a range of medicine may appear presumptuous. I have leaned heavily on friends who are experts in their own specialist fields to check thoroughly the factual material in order that the book, though written in plain language, should be as medically accurate as possible. If I have dealt too lightly here or in too great detail there, please excuse me. But here is where you come in. If enough people like this book, one day it may be reprinted; it can be improved only if you tell me its weaknesses and omissions. Any constructive criticism will be heeded and I will be thankful for it.

After reading the book put it in your rucksack, get out on the hills and enjoy yourself safely. Let us hope it stays in the sack, but should you need it take heart and remember you are not alone. I hope it will help you mobilize good sense into swift action.

Peter Steele. Bristol 1975.

Acknowledgements

These Bristol friends have given technical criticism of appropriate parts of this book, and I am deeply grateful for their labour and expertise:

Peter Baskett — Anaesthetist,
Monica Cooper — Medical Student,
Brian Cummins — Neurosurgeon,
Irene Fleming — Mother-in-law,
Harry Griffiths — Orthopaedic Surgeon,
Geoffrey Howden — Dental Surgeon,
Jo Leverment — Chest Surgeon,
Roy May — Abdominal Surgeon,
Ron Pigott — Plastic Surgeon,
John Verrier Jones — Physician,

and Sarah Steele, who loves me despite it all.

1

Casualty Assessment

At an accident in the mountains a climber is faced with a situation very different from emergencies that occur on the road, on the factory floor or at home, where ambulances are available to whisk the casualty to hospital. Distance from a road, difficult terrain and bad weather, all increase the time needed to reach skilled medical help. As climber-turned-doctor you are thrown on your own resources. You must gauge the seriousness of the victim's injury with your limited medical knowledge and try to prevent him dying or being further injured before you get help. This is a lonely and anxious time and, because of the sight of blood and a very sick casualty, you tend to panic. Most of us know the sickening empty feeling when faced with a predicament far beyond our previous experience. You need a cool head to assess the casualty's injuries, to judge the priorities and to take immediate appropriate action. When life is in imminent danger you must act promptly before trying to identify the precise reason for the trouble — contrary to usual medical practice which is to make an accurate diagnosis before starting treatment.

Move the casualty as little as possible to avoid causing him pain and so worsening his condition; but if he is lying in an awkward or dangerous place on the mountainside you may have to find level ground in order to revive him safely. Undo his helmet strap, which can interfere with breathing, and inspect his head for injury. If weather permits, loosen clothing round his neck and open his shirt so you can examine the whole of his chest; it is useless to pull clothes from his waist into a crumpled heap under his chin, and to lift them over his head may be impossible. If you suspect a chest injury or a broken limb and there are no buttons or a zip, cut down the seams and leave the clothes in place to keep the arms and back of the casualty warm and insulated from the ground.

A quick but careful scrutiny of the casualty should reveal his main injuries or problems; a full and leisurely examination can follow once you have answered this most urgent question:

"IS THE INJURED CLIMBER IN IMMEDIATE DANGER OF DYING?"

If he is, you must act fast and think later in order to keep him alive.

The scheme 'Ask/Look/Listen/Feel/Move/Act/Comfort/Carry' is a rough framework for most of the chapters in this book. 'How?' explains the background to the problem.

FIRST ASSESSMENT

Ask.

If the patient is fully conscious ask where he has pain and whether he can feel and move his limbs; otherwise gauge the conscious level by his response to question and command.

Look.

a. Appearance. Observe his general demeanour, whether he is lying still or rolling around. Note the colour of his face, especially the lips.

b. Breathing. Watch for movement of his chest.

c. Bleeding. Blood may be seen coming from an exposed wound. Blood-soaked clothing should be removed so you can see where bleeding is coming from. Look at the casualty's back and behind his head, where blood may have pooled unnoticed.

d. Pupils. Note the size of the pupils and whether they react to a light shone into them.

Listen.

Listen for the gentle sound of breathing at the mouth and the stertorous noise of airway block.

Feel.

Feel the radial pulse at the wrist and the carotid pulse in the neck. Gently feel the patient's neck, chest, abdomen, pelvis and limbs looking at his face all the time to see if light touch causes him to wince, indicating the site of his injury.

Move.

Ask the casualty to move his limbs by himself and only after he has tried to do so may you gently move them for him.

The injured climber is most likely to die from:

1. Inability to breathe due to airway block or chest injury.
2. Severe head injury and the sequels of unconsciousness.
3. Profuse bleeding which may cause shock and heart stop.

Act.

Do whatever you think necessary to prevent him dying from these causes and then take plenty of time for a careful and detailed assessment of the problem.

Comfort.

Make the patient comfortable and treat his pain with adequate doses of pain-killing analgesic drugs.

Carry.

Arrange to evacuate the casualty from the mountain in the manner you consider most suitable to his injury and circumstance.

Unless you are very far from help it is probably better to wait for the rescue team to arrive than to try to carry the casualty off the mountain in a make-shift stretcher.

The subject of mountain rescue is dealt with fully in the following books:—
The handbook of the Mountain Rescue Committee
International Mountain Rescue Handbook — Hamish MacInnes (Constable)

For general information about legion aspects of mountains consult:—
Mountaineering — Alan Blackshaw (Penguin)
Mountain Leadership — Eric Langmuir (Scottish Sports Council)

2

Airway Block

Breathing may appear to have stopped, but look carefully for shallow, quiet, normal breathing. Listen for a soft whistling noise at the casualty's mouth. In a cold climate the glass of a wristwatch or compass held close to his mouth may show hazy condensation of moist breath settling on the glass.

When the airway is partially blocked breathing is usually noisy, like someone snoring or croaking. The casualty's lips have a blue tinge (cyanosis) instead of their normal bright pink colour, and froth may appear in his mouth. Watch his chest carefully to see if it moves; if breathing is obstructed, chest movement is shallow and the spaces between the ribs are sucked inwards with each breath. By placing your ear against the casualty's chest you can hear sounds of breathing just as well as by using a stethoscope.

How?

The common causes of airway block are:—

1. The tongue falls back across the airway.
2. Saliva, blood or vomit pools in the airway.

a. Structure. The airway is the passage that conducts fresh air to the lungs. The nose and mouth are two cavities separated by the palate beyond which a common passage, the pharynx, is formed. The soft palate makes a flap-valve that closes off the nose from the back of the mouth and prevents regurgitation. Air passes between the vocal cords of the larynx into the trachea (windpipe), and into the bronchi, which divide like the branches of a tree into narrower and narrower tubes, bronchioles and alveoli. The larynx guards the entrance to the lungs; on breathing in, the vocal cords move apart, returning to the half-way position on breathing out. During swallowing, the vocal cords and soft parts of the larynx close tightly to prevent any foreign matter entering the lungs.

In quiet normal breathing air passes through the nose; the mouth remains closed, almost completely filled by the tongue which lies well forwards against the teeth and the hard palate. It is vital to know the structure and function of the tongue in order to understand the principles of airway block.

The tongue is a large muscle, fixed at its base to the mandible (lower jaw). Only about one third of its total bulk is seen when fully protruded. The tongue of a conscious person is kept forwards in the mouth by active muscle effort; while he is lying face upwards, asleep or unconscious, all his muscles relax and the tongue falls back by gravity. This partly shuts off the airway and causes the characteristic sound of snoring, when the partially relaxed tongue vibrates against the back of the throat as air slips past. An unconscious person loses control of his tongue muscle, and when fully relaxed it forms an almost air-tight obstruction, like a cork, across the pharynx.

Airway block caused by the tongue is most commonly seen in persons who are unconscious from head or chest injuries, or from severe blood loss. Saliva, blood or vomit may also cause a partial block which, if it becomes complete, will suffocate the casualty.

Coughing, swallowing and closing the larynx are defence reflexes, under nervous control, that prevent food, water and vomit ‘going down the wrong way’ into

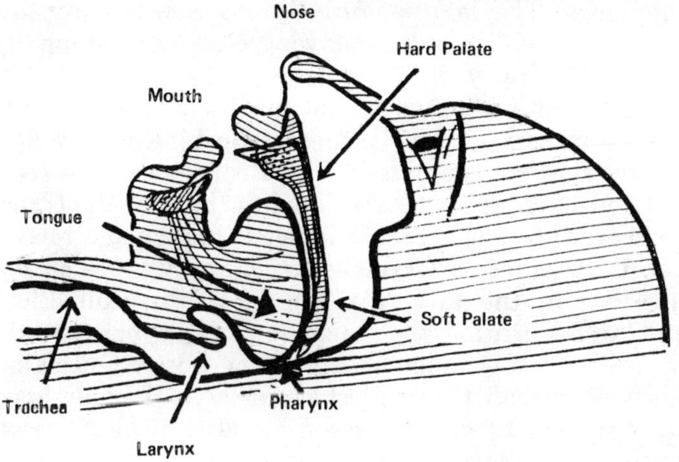

Figure 2.1 Airway block due to the tongue

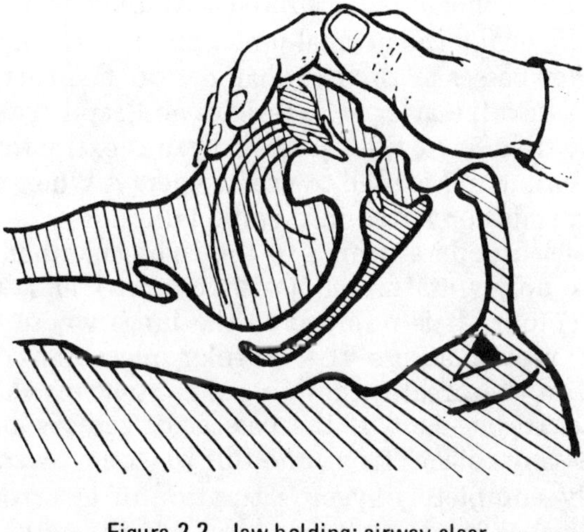

Figure 2.2 Jaw holding; airway clear

the lungs. The larynx normally closes when someone vomits; coughing and swallowing clear any vomit that enters the airway.

The vomiting reflex of an unconscious person may still be present but the laryngeal, coughing and swallowing reflexes are suppressed. Saliva continues to be secreted and blood may trickle down the back of the throat, so these substances can be inhaled through the relaxed vocal cords into the trachea and on into the smaller divisions of the lung tree, causing obstruction. Blood and vomit irritate the lining mucosa, which secretes more fluid, so making the problem worse. Once fluid lies in the alveoli, the smallest air passages, the membrane for exchange of gases between blood and the air ceases to function properly.

b. Function. Inhaled air contains 20 per cent oxygen, which passes across the one-cell-thick wall of the lung alveolus into the venous blood and is taken up by haemoglobin in the red blood cells. This (unsaturated) venous blood becomes saturated with oxygen and turns bright red, giving the normal pink colour to the lips. The blood then passes to the left chamber of the heart which pumps it into the arteries, arterioles and capillaries of all the body tissues. At the tissues oxygen is extracted from arterial blood and is used to create energy. When burned up, oxygen is converted into carbon dioxide.

Venous blood returning to the right chamber of the heart is now unsaturated (with oxygen) and a deep purple colour. It is pumped to the lungs where carbon dioxide moves across the alveolar membrane and is exhaled in the breath, the oxygen content of which has fallen to 16 per cent. If the passage of gases is interrupted, at any place from mouth to lung alveoli, the normally complete oxygen saturation of arterial blood is diminished and pink lips turn bluish or cyanotic.

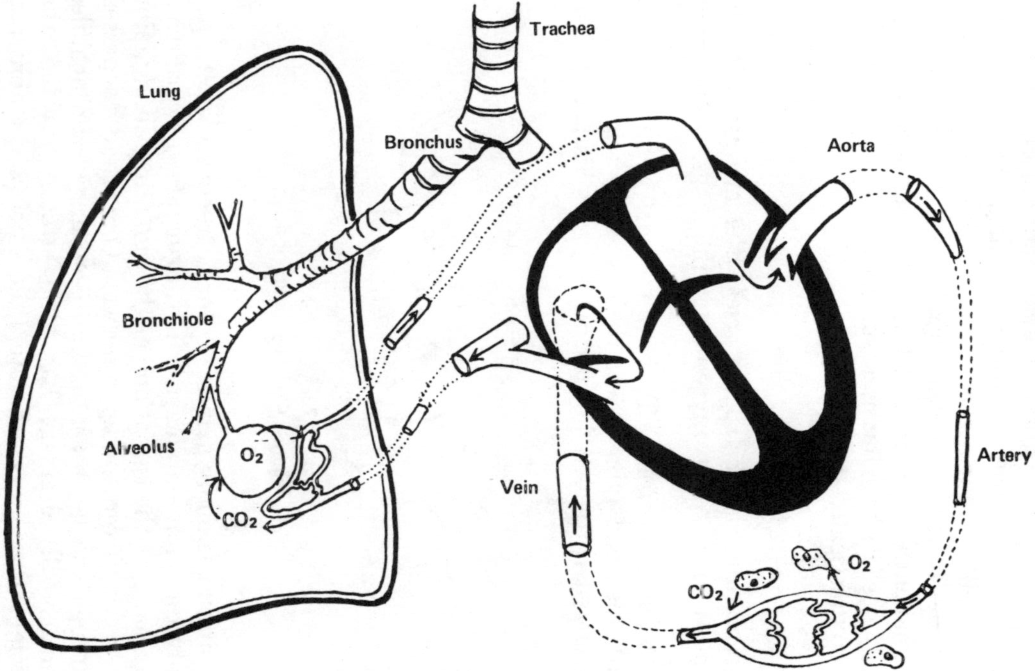

Figure 2.3 Heart and lung structure and function

After more than four minutes without oxygen the brain suffers irreparable damage and more and more cells die the longer oxygen is lacking. Dead brain and nerve cells cannot regenerate and although the casualty may partly recover consciousness later, his brain will be permanently damaged. All tissues and organs of the body need oxygen but none suffers deprivation so quickly or so drastically as the brain.

Act.

If breathing is obstructed, clear the airway with the utmost speed to let oxygen reach the lungs.

1. Draining position. Turn the casualty on one side with his head lying lower than his body and the neck extended (provided he has not injured his neck). This

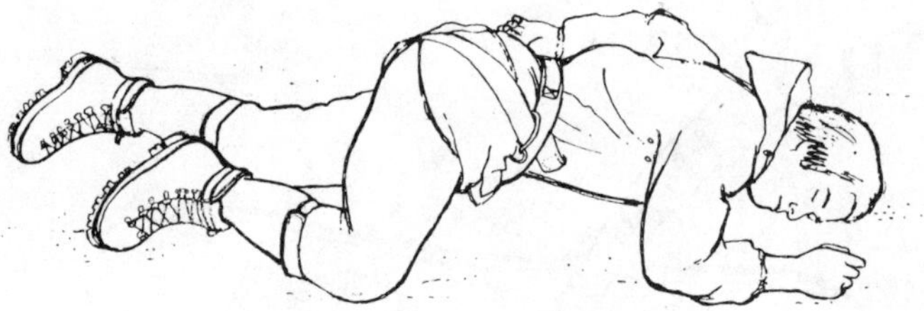

Figure 2.4 The draining position

position has many names, 'coma', 'recovery', etc., but only one aim — drainage. The tongue falls forward from the back of the throat and at the same time fluid drains by gravity from the upper airway. Once fluid has passed through the larynx into the lower airway (bronchioles and alveoli) drainage has little effect. Provided the patient does not suffocate fluid is slowly reabsorbed into the blood stream, as happens in near-drowning. So turn him into the draining position with all speed.

2. Secretions. Having removed any dentures put your finger, wrapped with a piece of cloth, into the casualty's mouth and scoop or mop out solid matter such as vomited food, blood clot, or avalanche powder-snow. Someone emerging from coma may clench his teeth tight so you cannot force his jaws apart. If he relaxes try to put a wedge (a rolled handkerchief or a piece of wood) between his teeth to prevent him biting his tongue — and your fingers. A person close to dying will eventually relax, but by then it may be too late.

The most effective way of removing fluid from the airway is to suck it out. Pass a soft flexible tube far back in the throat, suck on it and spit out the material. If secretions pooled near the larynx are causing obstruction this unpleasant task may be life-saving.

Foot-operated suction pumps should be available in all resuscitation kits carried by rescue services.

3. Jaw holding. If the jaw is held forward correctly the tongue moves with it and cannot fall back against the pharynx to block the airway, because the root of the tongue arises from and is fixed to the mandible (lower jaw). The crucial difference between pulling the lower jaw forwards and merely closing the upper and lower teeth together can be appreciated by understanding the mechanics of the mandibular joint.

The lower jaw has rounded ends that fit into hollows on the under-side of the skull and rock backwards and forwards. The opening jaw slides forwards over a small hump and lies in a shallow groove 1 cm. in front of the main joint surface. You can feel this sliding action if you place your fingers in front of your ear lobes and thrust your jaw forwards. This displacement prevents the posterior part of the tongue falling back across the airway.

Holding the jaw incorrectly can be dangerous, as you may close the mouth with the tongue still lying back.

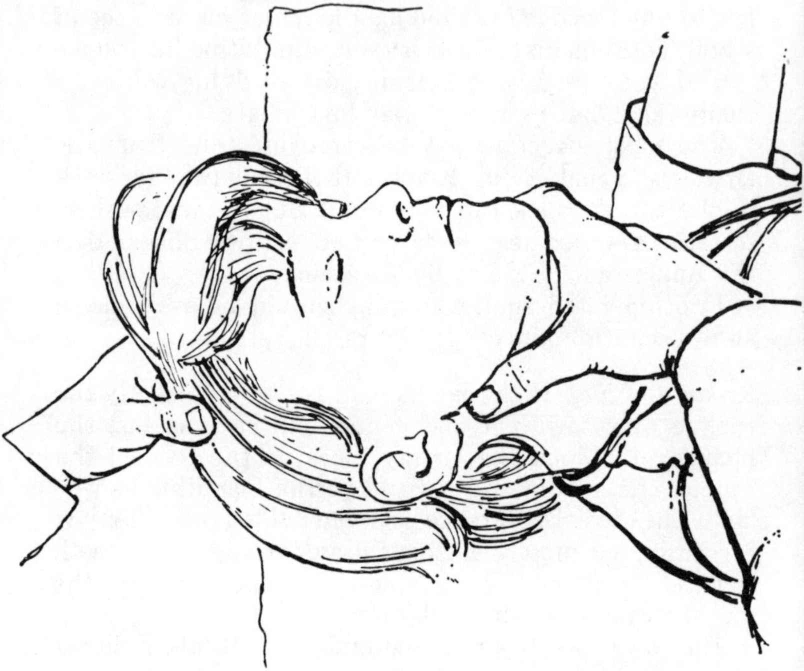

Figure 2.5a Jaw holding

Although it is easier to hold the jaw forward with the casualty lying on his back, you should be able to do it in the draining position. The casualty's neck should be straight to prevent the trachea kinking.

With your three middle fingers widely spaced grasp the casualty's jaw, one hand on each side. The key to efficient jaw-holding is the little finger, which is curled behind the angle of the jaw and then pushes upwards towards the sky. This moves the whole jaw forwards into the groove on the base of the skull. By resting your elbows on the ground you can maintain this tiring position for longer. If the casualty is lying on his side in the draining position, your hands hold the jaw in exactly the same way.

Anaesthetists, who are skilled and constantly practised in airway control, often hold the point of the jaw with one hand to leave the other hand free, but this

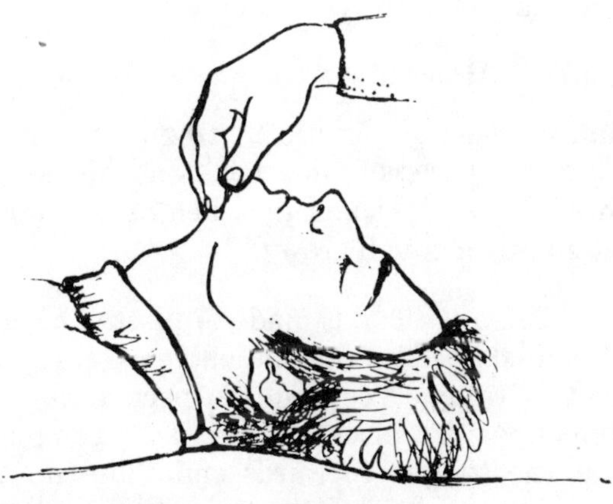

Figure 2.5b Jaw holding (expert)

method requires practice and is only for experts.

If you remember that the tongue is attached to the jaw then airway control becomes a logical exercise.

4. Tongue fixing. If you cannot keep the chin forward and the tongue persistently falls back (e.g. while carrying the casualty on a stretcher) thrust a safety-pin right through the tip of his tongue, tie a piece of string or cord to it and pull firmly forwards; this apparently brutal action does little damage to the tongue and guarantees a clear airway.

Persistent airway block. If the casualty's breathing remains obstructed despite adequate:—

1. Drainage,
2. Suction,
3. Chin holding,
4. Tongue fixing,

— then mechanical 'airways' are necessary.

A. Mechanical 'Airways'

A mechanical 'airway' is useful when an unconscious casualty's tongue keeps falling back and his jaw is difficult to hold forward, especially when he is being carried on a stretcher over rough ground.

1. Guedel 'Airway'. This is made of plastic, hard rubber or metal, and shaped so the end curves over the back of the casualty's tongue keeping the space at the back of the pharynx open. To insert the 'airway' open his mouth wide, pull the tongue forwards and slide the 'airway' over it into place. A wet 'airway' slides in place more easily. The tooth guard prevents a half-conscious patient

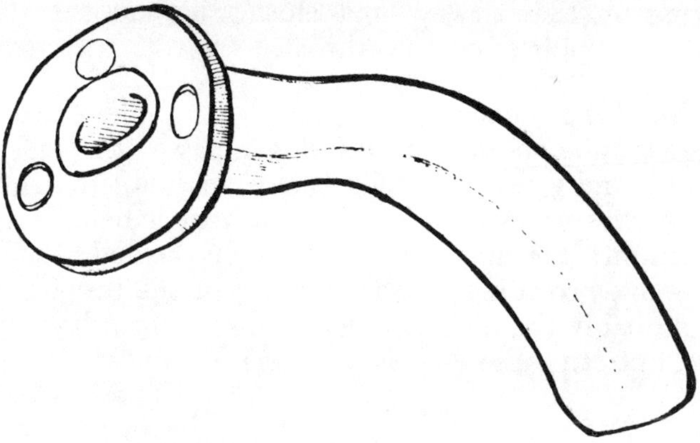

Figure 2.6 Guedel 'airway'

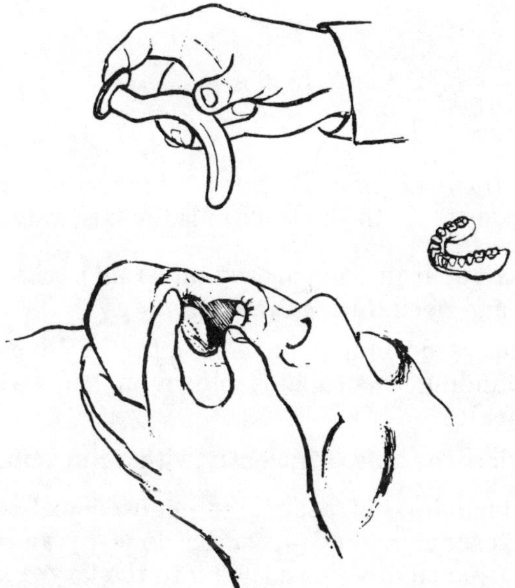

Figure 2.7 Guedel 'airway' insertion

biting on the 'airway' and closing it, and the flange stops it slipping down his throat.

2. *Nasal (naso-pharyngeal) 'Airway'.* A well greased soft rubber tube about 6 inches long is passed through one nostril and gently threaded backwards until the rubber flange lies against the nose (to prevent it being sucked down into the lung). In this position the end lies in the pharynx providing a clear airway past the tongue. This is probably the most efficient 'airway' for a layman to use, but can cause damage if done roughly.

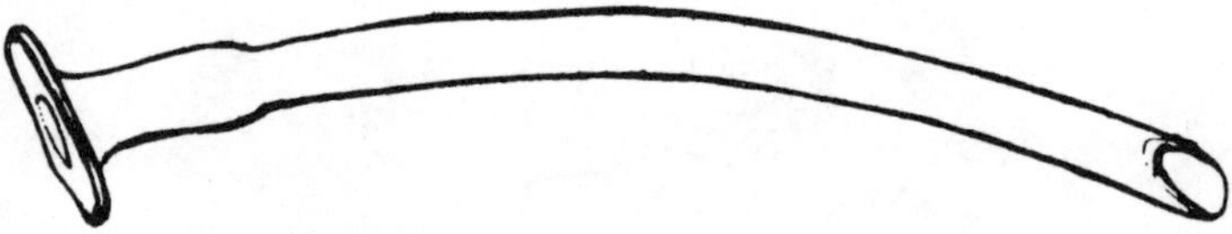

Figure 2.8 Nasal airway

3. *Endotracheal tube.* Passing a plastic tube through the vocal cords to lie in the trachea is the best way:—

a. to guarantee an open airway under all positions of the head and neck during evacuation;
b. to ensure nothing is inhaled into the lungs, (a cuff surrounding the tube is blown up to seal off the trachea);
c. to inflate the lungs efficiently with a resuscitation bag.

The technique of passing an endotracheal tube using a laryngoscope should *never* be done by an untrained person. Clumsily forcing a tube into the larynx can make the vocal cords go into spasm, and they may only relax just before the casualty is about to die of airway obstruction.

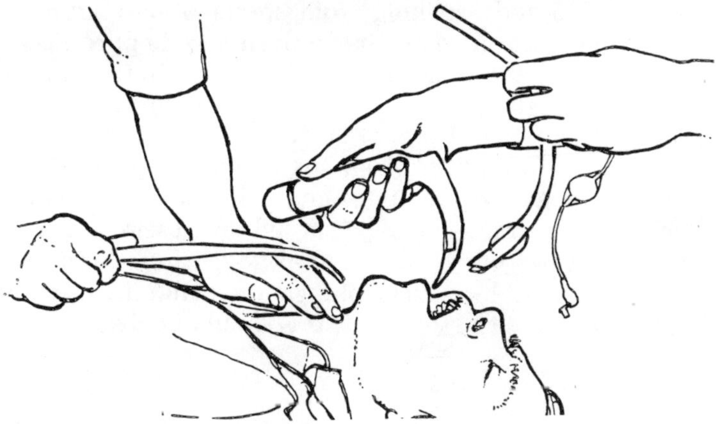

Figure 2.9 Passing an endotracheal tube

Intubation is usually carried out by doctors, and anaesthetists in particular, but it involves no special mystique. It is a skill that has to be acquired, and, like riding a bicycle, once learned is never forgotten. There is no reason why mountain rescue team members should not learn to intubate a casualty; nowadays in some enlightened centres ambulance men are taught by an anaesthetist at their local hospital. But the technique requires several weeks of intensive practice and cannot be learned quickly in one afternoon.

4. Tracheostomy. Tracheostomy is a surgical operation whereby a hole is cut through the skin of the neck, below the Adam's apple (cartilage of the larynx) into the trachea, bypassing the airway above the vocal cords. Tracheostomy should be done in hospital as it is difficult to perform. Under emergency situations such as on a mountain it is easier and safer to pass a well-greased endotracheal tube which can be left in position safely for 48 hours or more. However, when a casualty is blue in the face and croaking from spasm of the larynx, a life-saving measure may be to push a wide-bore needle directly into the trachea through the skin in the midline of the neck about $1\frac{1}{2}''$ (3 cm.) below the prominence of the Adam's apple. A hiss of air is released as it enters the trachea. A few puffs of air (or better oxygen) may be enough to aerate the lungs and relax the vocal cords. But Needle tracheostomy should be reserved for an extreme emergency only, and although lives have been saved by skilful rescuers plunging a penknife into the neck with a twist of the wrist, this should be discouraged.

B. Assisted Breathing

If, despite a patent airway, the patient is not breathing, then artificial ventilation to blow vital oxygen into the lungs is urgently necessary.

The aim of assisted breathing is to move air into the lungs, letting the natural elasticity of both the lungs and the rib cage expel it. Although not as good as pure air,

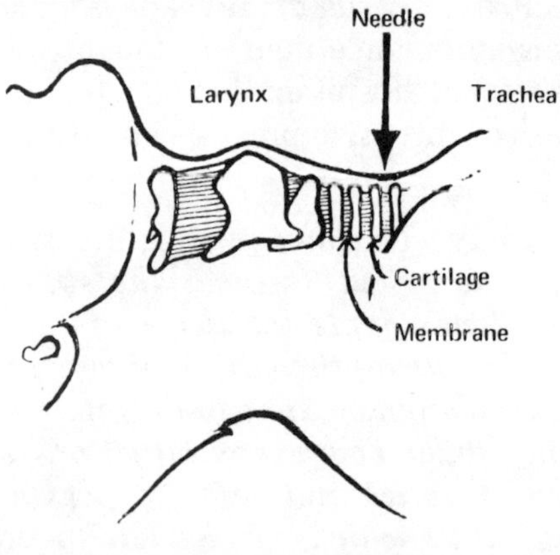

Figure 2.10 Needle tracheostomy

your own nasty expired breath still contains 16 per cent oxygen, which is enough to change a casualty's colour from blue to pink. Keep watching the patient's chest to see that your assisted breathing is being effective.

a. Mouth-to-mouth (the unsavoury 'kiss of life'). Turn the casualty on his back because mouth-to-mouth breathing is difficult to carry out if he is lying on his side. Tip back his head which straightens the neck, in order (a) to keep the airway open, and (b) to prevent air passing down the oesophagus (gullet) and so inflating the stomach. After wiping away any debris place your mouth over that of the casualty and pinch his nose to stop air escaping. If you place an open handkerchief across his mouth the procedure is less distasteful.

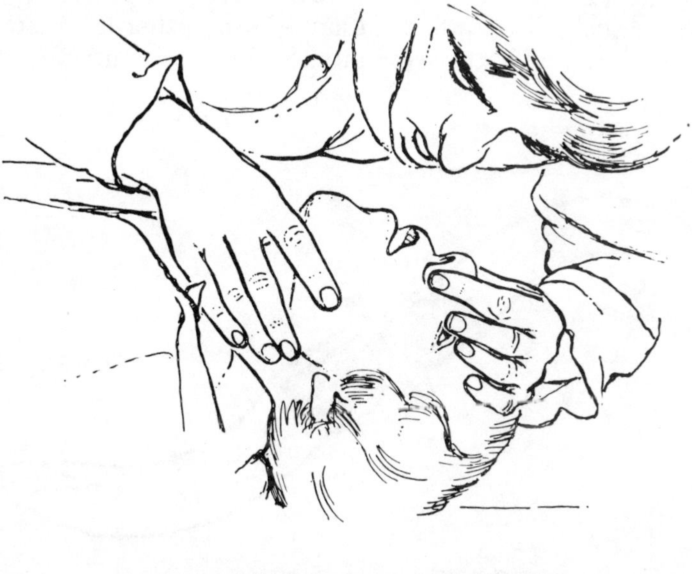

Figure 2.11 Mouth-to-mouth assisted breathing

Watch his chest rise as the lungs are inflated; about $\frac{1}{4}$-$\frac{1}{2}$ litre of air should be shifted with each breath. Then remove your mouth and the elasticity of the patient's own lungs will expel the air. One breath every 4-6 seconds is ample. If the casualty's mouth is injured you may have to breathe into his nose instead, holding his lips closed while doing this. Mouth-to-mouth breathing is far more efficient than any of the mechanical methods of 'artificial respiration' that used to be taught by life-savers; these routines move much less air than mouth-to-mouth breathing and are complicated, so you may forget the urgent importance of shifting air in and out of the lungs.

The following more elaborate mechanical 'airways' make mouth-to-mouth breathing more efficient and less unpleasant for the rescuer.

i. The two-ended Guedel 'Airway'. One end passes into the casualty's mouth as described, the other is free to blow into and so to avoid mouth-to-mouth contact (see

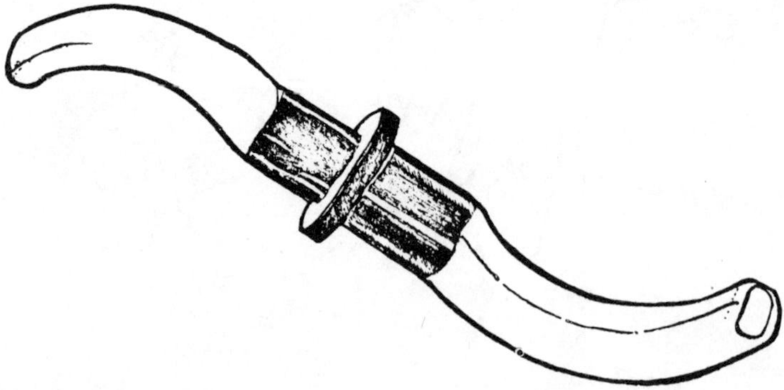

Figure 2.12 Two-ended Guedel 'airway'

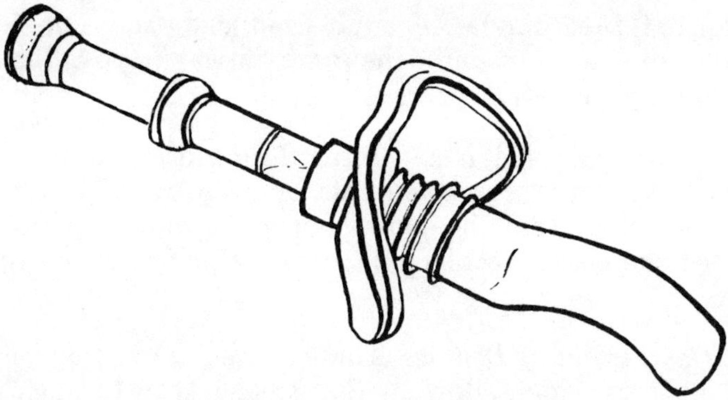

Figure 2.13 Brook 'airway'

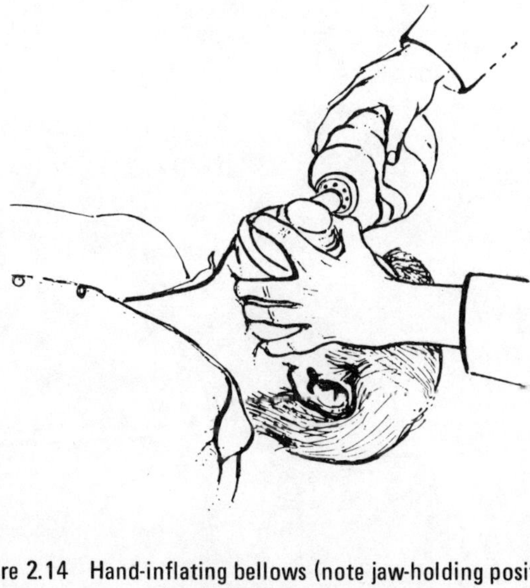

Figure 2.14 Hand-inflating bellows (note jaw-holding position)

Assisted Breathing). An adult-sized end, and one for children can be made in the same 'airway', providing a dual-purpose tool.

ii. Brook 'Airway'. A cheek guard fits closely round the casualty's mouth and a simple one-way valve prevents air escaping from the lungs. When the mouth guard is lifted the elastic recoil of the casualty's chest expels the air.

b. Hand Inflating Bellows. These are self-expanding bags or bellows which allow air that is sucked in through a valve at one end to be expelled at the other. Inflation is easier work and can be continued for longer than mouth-to-mouth breathing. The bellows can either be attached to a face mask that fits over the nose and mouth, or to a tube that connects it with an endotracheal tube.

3

Heart Stop

There are three reliable signs that the heart has stopped; (all three must be present for the diagnosis to be made).

1. Unconsciousness

2. Absent pulse

3. Colour change

Usually breathing stops at the same time and the airway must be cleared and assisted breathing given as described earlier, in order to get oxygen to the lungs.

1. Unconsciousness.

The patient does not respond to command or pain. The pupils of the eyes slowly widen and do not contract to a pin-point when a light is shone into them.

2. Pulse.

Feeling the pulse at the wrist is notoriously misleading, and the rescuer searching for it with cold hands and with a casualty's tight elastic anorak cuffs, may get a false impression that the heart has stopped. Feel in the neck for the pulsation of the carotid artery where pressure is high, being only a short distance from the heart. Place three fingers alongside the trachea (windpipe) and press steadily for several seconds, with your eyes closed to help concentration. If still in doubt listen with your ear pressed close to the left side of the casualty's chest. The heart sounds like a distant "lub-dup, lub-dup, lub-dup".

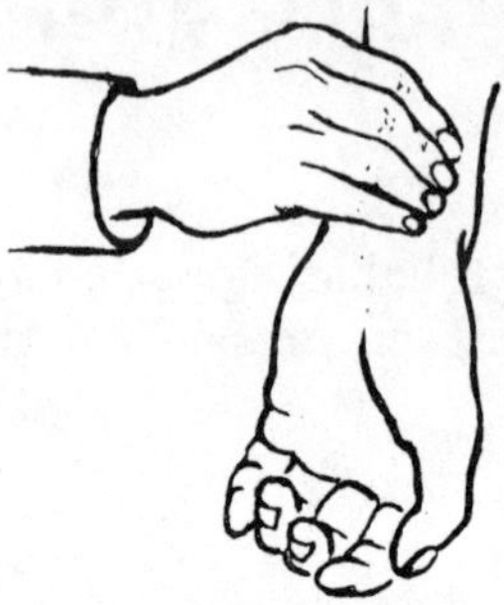

Figure 3.1 Feeling the wrist pulse

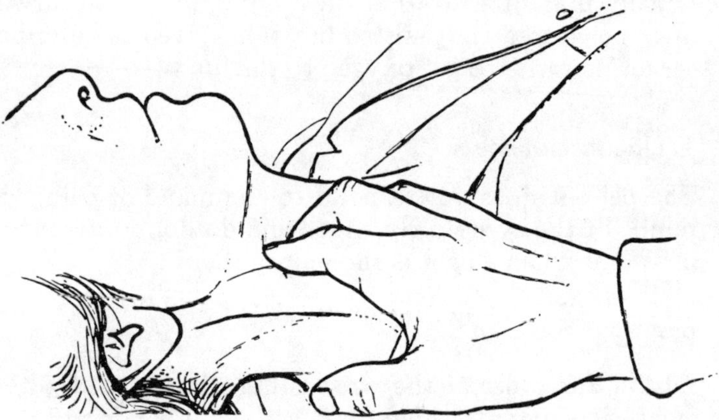

Figure 3.2 Feeling the carotid pulse

3. Colour.

The skin of a collapsed person, especially of the hands and feet, is usually cold and bloodless, so its colour does not reflect accurately the state of the heart. The reason for this is (a) his blood vessels are constricted, which is Nature's way of keeping the blood volume in the central core of the body where it is needed for the function of the vital organs (brain, heart, lungs and kidneys), (b) he may be cold because of the temperature in the outside environment. Examine the colour of the lips and the mucous membrane inside the mouth, best seen by pulling down the lower lip; when the heart has stopped the colour will be blue or very pale instead of the usual pink.

Act.

If the heart and breathing have been stopped for less than four minutes you must take urgent action. If the victim has been "dead" for more than 15 minutes attempts at rescue are futile. In the between time you have to use your discretion.

Another rescuer should start assisted breathing immediately. A sharp blow with a clenched fist on the lower part of the casualty's chest may be enough to restart his heart. If this does not succeed begin chest compression (external heart massage). Lay the casualty flat on a hard surface. Compress the heart between the sternum (breastbone) and the spine, using the elasticity of the ribs as a springboard. The spine projects well forwards into the chest, the distance between it and the sternum being only about 5 inches (10 cm.). Raise the casualty's legs above the level of his body, by resting his feet on a rucksack, in order to drain blood from the veins of his legs into his central circulation. Kneel beside him and place the heel of one of your hands over the lower part of his breastbone and with your other hand press on the one below. Rock forwards and backwards on your hips with your arms straight, pressing down hard on his chest and then relaxing, once each second.

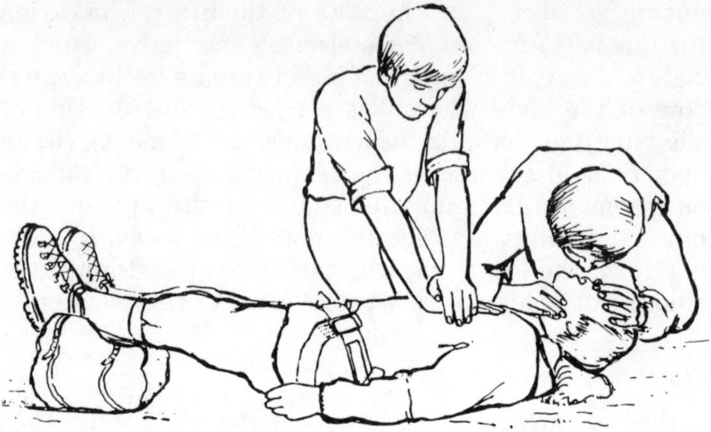

Figure 3.3 Chest compression – PRESS

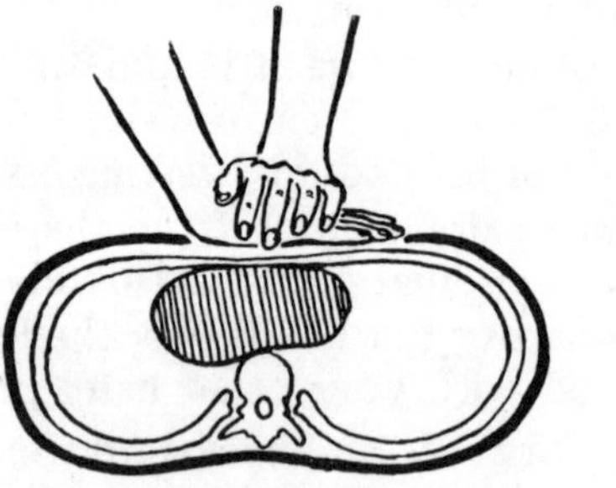

Figure 3.4 Chest compression (insert of X-sec)

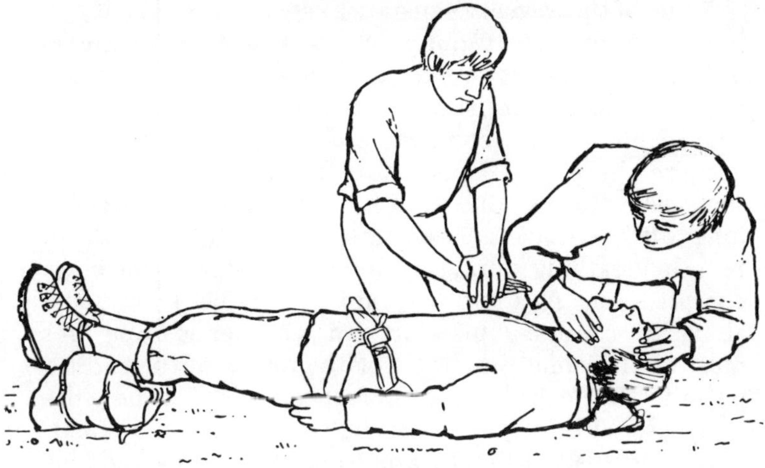

Figure 3.5 Chest compression — REST

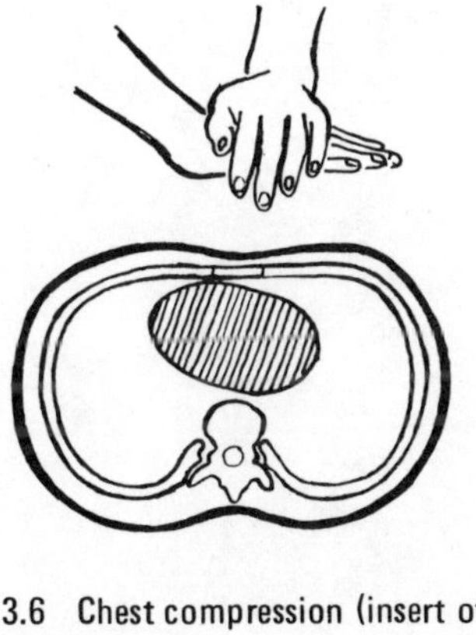

Figure 3.6 Chest compression (insert of X-sec)

Some of the casualty's ribs are likely to be broken if you press hard enough to pump his heart adequately. This is not as serious as it sounds and can be dealt with later. Chest compression is very exhausting so you should change places with someone else every five minutes. If you are alone, give 4 pumps to the casualty's heart and then pause to give one mouth-to-mouth inflation of his lungs. If you have an assistant, he can give mouth-to-mouth breathing during a moment's pause from heart compression. Assisted breathing must be kept going alongside chest compression and whoever is doing this must at the same time feel for the return of the carotid pulse in the neck. In order to feel carefully for the pulse all resuscitation may have to be stopped for a moment.

If the casualty's heart starts to beat on its own and his breathing continues unassisted, he will become warmer, a pink colour replaces the blueness of the lips and pallor of the skin and mucous membranes, and the large dilated pupils return to their normal size aperture. Continue to watch the casualty closely because the heart and breathing may suddenly stop. You must then begin resuscitating him again.

4

Head Injury

A climber may strike his head during a tumble or be hit by falling rock or ice from the mountain above. Hard protective helmets have become accepted and, like motor cycle crash-hats and car seat-belts, have reduced the serious effects of head injuries. Whereas climbing helmets were rarely seen on the rocks twenty years ago, nowadays climbers not using them are considered foolhardy.

At the scene of an accident where a climber has injured his head you must act immediately to prevent him dying from:—

1. Airway block (see Chapter 2)

A climber with a severe head injury will usually be unconscious. If he is lying on his back his tongue falls backwards blocking his airway. He may also be in danger of inhaling blood from an associated face injury.

2. Severe bleeding (see Chapter 5)

The scalp and face bleed freely; although alarming, this loss of blood alone is a poor indication of the gravity of a head injury. Press firmly over the wound with a dressing pad until bleeding stops, then cover the wound with a dry dressing and a firm crepe bandage. If you find an open skull wound or suspect a depressed fracture place a ring pad so the ring rests on undamaged skull and the centre lies over the wound, causing no pressure.

After making sure the airway is clear and bleeding has

stopped, your most important task in caring for a climber with a head injury is to observe him carefully and make an accurate record of your findings *in writing.* If his brain has been damaged the neurosurgeon, who will see him for the first time some hours later, will be grateful for your observations of the changing trends in the patient's condition, on which he bases his diagnosis. On the mountain you can do no more than prevent the casualty dying from other causes before he reaches skilled help.

How?

The brain is the nerve centre of the body. Brain is composed of semi-solid matter suspended in cerebro-spinal fluid which cushions its movement within a rigid protective box, the skull. Cerebro-spinal fluid circulates between a layer of arachnoid tissue, which covers the brain, and another of dura, which lies against the skull. Blood vessels lying in the space between brain and arachnoid, and between skull and dura, are liable to be torn in a head injury. The released blood has no means of escape and collects in spaces between the covering layers. If bleeding is profuse, pressure inside the skull rises, damaging the delicate nerve cells of the brain.

Injury to the brain is determined by the type of force applied to the head. A piece of fractured skull may pierce the brain directly under the point of impact; the brain may swirl inside the skull so that soft fibre pathways shear off each other causing many small bleeding points. The brain may rebound from the impact squashing itself against the opposite wall of the skull (contrecoup). Released blood may be unable to escape, or the brain may swell so the casualty is at first conscious but confused, and then lapses into coma.

Brain damage may be local or diffuse, and its severity will determine the state of the injured climber.

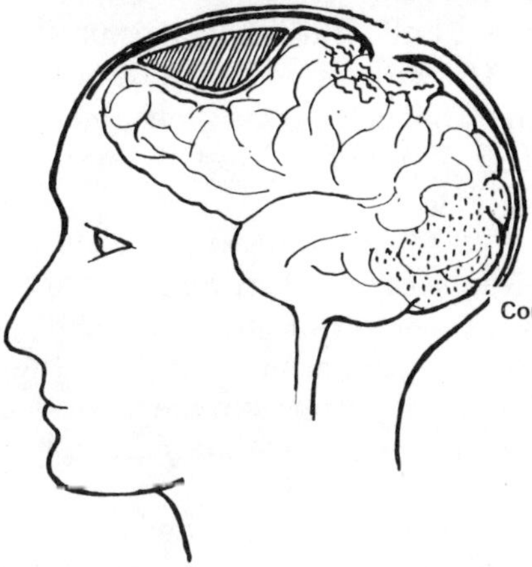

Figure 4.1 Brain injuries

A simple guide to the types of brain damage is:—

1. Concussion — trivial injury causes brief unconsciousness and confusion = Speedy complete recovery.
2. Local Damage — epileptic fits occur with frequent lapses of consciousness, jerking and occasionally paralysis of the limbs on the opposite side of the body = Slow recovery.
3. Clot Compression — after being knocked-out the casualty first improves (lucid interval), then he slides quickly into unconsciousness = Death unless pressure is relieved.
4. Severe Diffuse Injury — the victim is unconscious from the time of the fall. He is incapable of maintaining his airway, which may become blocked = Very slow recovery over months.

1. Concussion (knock-out). A blow on the head may not damage the skull but the deceleration force causes the brain to swirl round inside it, nerve pathways are deranged and the person becomes unconscious. He may recover after a period of rest if there is no major damage to brain tissue.

Someone who has been 'knocked out' may be unconscious from a few seconds to several minutes. He may forget the impact itself but will probably remember events up to a definite moment *before* the accident which are followed by a measurable period of forgetfulness or 'blank' (retrograde amnesia); as he improves this period may shrink.

The blank period *after* an accident (post-traumatic amnesia) is a guide to the degree of seriousness of the head injury and indicates the speed at which recovery may be expected.

i.e.	less than one hour	— mild head injury = rapid complete recovery.
	one hour to one day	— moderate head injury = recovery over weeks.
	one day to seven days	— severe head injury = recovery over months.
	more than one week	— very severe head injury = full recovery unlikely.

This blank period is important because the injured climber may feel fine after the accident and set off down the mountain alone, having no recollection of what happened to him or of his whereabouts. He may lose his path, or worse, relapse on the way down and collapse on the open mountain due to pressure from slow hidden bleeding building up inside the skull. Anyone who has lost consciousness from a head injury, for however short a time, should not be allowed to descend unaided even if he feels confident that his injury was trivial.

2. *Local damage.* The brain has well-defined areas looking after particular functions such as moving each limb, controlling speech and perceiving sensation. The right half of the brain controls the left side of the body, the left side of the brain the right side of the body. Local damage may cause paralysis or, if not so severe, irritation of the brain with fits of twitching of the opposite limbs. It is most important to observe and record these 'local' fits. They may spread into general 'grand mal' fits, during which the injured person may die unless the airway is closely guarded.

3. *Clot compression (pressure on the brain).* A trifling knock on the head is commonly followed by a period of concussion. The victim may appear quite normal a short while later and may even continue climbing. This time of apparent normality before relapse is called the 'lucid interval'. Then the casualty begins to 'go off', gradually and often unnoticeably, and he becomes steadily more drowsy until he slips into coma. These are the classic signs of bleeding within the skull and rising pressure on the brain, which is one of the most urgent emergencies in medicine. Continued bleeding or swelling of the brain itself causes pressure within the rigid skull to rise because there is little room for expansion. If this pressure is not released, damage to the brain is inevitable and permanent. The cells of the cortex (outer layer of the brain) die and do not regrow unlike cells in other parts of the body.

The victim will die if the pressure is not quickly released by trephining a hole in the skull. Surgery is the only treatment, so all the rescuers can do is to evacuate the victim fast.

4. Severe diffuse injury. The climber will be deeply unconscious and quite unable to help himself. He may be lax or stiff. Unless prevented, he may roll about in a purposeless manner and fall again. If you can take good care of his airway he may make a first rate recovery.

Observations

Write down careful and accurate observations at least every half hour. If you do not write all your notes it is unlikely you will remember the exact sequence and timing in the tumult of the rescue. These notes may show any progressing trends of improvement or deterioration in a patient's behaviour and will help a surgeon distinguish between simple concussion and rising pressure. This may make him decide to operate within minutes of the patient's arrival at the hospital.

Ask.

Try to get information about the accident either from the injured climber, if he is conscious, or from someone present at the time.

— What is the name, age, and address of the casualty? Does he carry a blood group card or other medical details?

— How did the accident occur? Was the climber roped, wearing a helmet and how far was the fall?

— Has the victim complained of headache starting some time after the accident?

— Has he had a fit after the injury?

— At what time did the accident occur? What was the casualty's last memory before, and the first memory after, the injury? This allows you to measure any retrograde or post-traumatic amnesia.

— Has the casualty's behaviour or level of consciousness

changed in any way?

Look.

1. Appearance of the head. Remove the climbing helmet and inspect the whole head carefully. Slip your hand under his head to see if blood has pooled there. Clean any wounds with soap and water and remove blood clot to show the base of the wound where you may find a fracture, or pieces of foreign material that must be removed before putting on a dressing. Never push instruments into a wound as you may introduce infection and even penetrate the brain through an open skull fracture.

When no open wound exists, a soft swelling under the scalp points to blood collecting at the site of a skull fracture. Blood or clear fluid coming from the nose or ears, when not caused by obvious external injury, suggests a fracture of the base of the skull with leakage of cerebro-spinal fluid or bleeding from the vessels over the surface of the brain.

Antibiotic treatment must be started immediately, using large doses of sulphadimidine and penicillin.

2. Conscious level. A head injury victim is likely to have been knocked out, however briefly; he may be unconscious when you see him or in the twilight of stupor, emerging from his blackout. Exact terms are needed to avoid confusion.

The conscious level of the casualty may be graded as follows:—

Level 1. Talks rationally. He is able to give a full account of the accident and remember being knocked out.

Level 2. Talks, but is confused. He is unable to remember the accident or to say who or where he is.

Level 3. Responds to simple commands. He is unable to talk but puts out his tongue on command.

Level 4. Responds to pain.

(a) actively. If you pinch his skin or squeeze his Achilles tendon he tries to push your hand away.

(b) passively. He withdraws from the offending stimulus. He does not blink when you stroke his eyelashes.

Level 5. Does not respond to pain. Damn near dead.

A changing conscious level shows that a casualty is becoming 'lighter' and approaching normal, or is becoming 'deeper' with increasing pressure on the brain and loss of reflexes. The trend will not show on a single examination, but may be obvious from your serial written observations.

If there is no bruise on the head and no witness to the accident, remember other causes of coma, as a person found unconscious on the mountain may not have suffered a head injury at all (see p. 130 for a fuller account).

— Epilepsy. He may bite his tongue, froth at the mouth, or twitch.

— Diabetes. Look for a medallion or bracelet that a diabetic may carry to warn you of his condition. His breath may have the sweet smell of pear drops (ketones).

— Alcohol. His breath gives the story away.

— Heart Attack. The victim is likely to be an older person who is shocked and short of breath.

3. *Pupils of the eyes.* If the brain is pressed on by an enlarging clot of blood the nerve that controls the size of the pupil becomes stretched and eventually paralysed. The

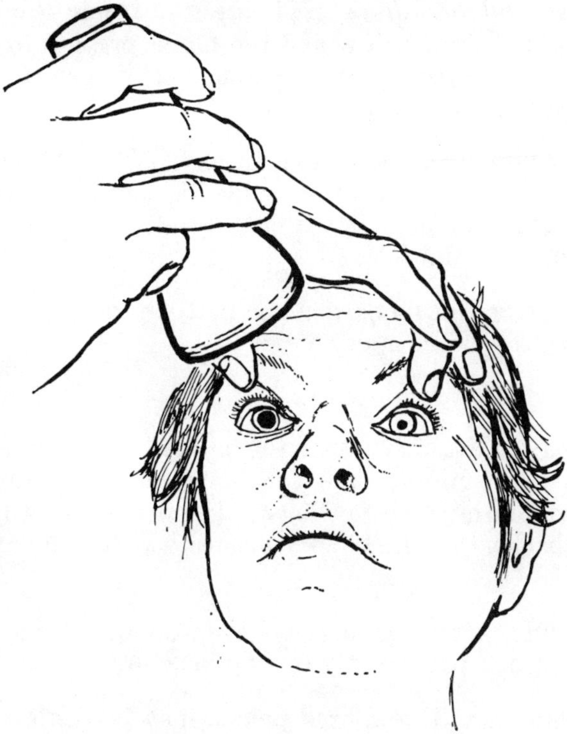

Figure 4.2 Pupil reaction to light

pupil on the same side as the clot enlarges, and fails to contract to a pin-point when the eye is opened to daylight or an electric torch is shone into it. This observation is crucial, as it will tell the surgeon in which side of the head he should drill his trephine hole. If the pressure is not relieved the pupil on the opposite side becomes paralysed. Two fixed dilated pupils is a very grave sign that recovery is unlikely.

4. Pulse and breathing. High pressure inside the skull causes the pulse to slow and the blood pressure to rise (N.B. opposite to shock). Breathing becomes stertorous, like snoring, and may be irregular.

5. Sensation. Loss of feeling in any part of the body indicates damage to the brain, spine, or peripheral nerves. Lightly touching the skin with a pin will show you where sensation is diminished.

6. Paralysis. The limbs may be partially or completely paralysed by brain injury.

Act.

a. Airway. First make sure the injured climber has no serious neck injury, then turn him into the draining position and hold his jaw forward to prevent his tongue falling backwards and blocking the airway. Remove false teeth.

b. Bleeding. After cleaning any head wound, cover it with a dressing and press firmly to stop bleeding.

c. Restlessness. The injured person may be restless and need restraining (possibly because of a full bladder). Drugs should not be used, especially those of the morphia family, since they depress breathing, alter the level of consciousness and make the pupils smaller, thereby disguising a vital observation.

d. Keep accurate written records and get the victim to hospital without delay. If he has been unconscious, however briefly, he should be checked by a doctor.

5

Haemorrhage and Shock

Bleeding (haemorrhage) must be stopped immediately by pressing firmly on the wound, raising the injured part, and putting the casualty at rest.

How?

An average adult male has about 10 pints ($5\frac{1}{2}$ litres) of circulating blood, a female about 8 pints ($4\frac{1}{2}$ litres). They can afford to lose about 2 pints (1 litre) before serious effects of anaemia and shock are noticed. Loss of more than a third of the body's blood volume can kill. A child has less blood in proportion to its size than an adult, so can tolerate losing only a small amount.

Blood left to stand in a test tube settles out in two layers; above is a straw-coloured fluid, plasma or serum, and below are red blood cells and other cells only visible with a microscope. If the tube is gently shaken the cells mix with the plasma in which they are suspended making an even red solution. After bleeding the number of red cells in the blood drops although the plasma is quickly made up from other body fluids. The blood is diluted and the person becomes anaemic, being pale, tired and weak. Lost red cells are normally replaced over a period of weeks by new cells being made in the bone marrow.

Blood flows through a complex plumbing system. The heart, though considered by some to be the seat of the soul, is little more than a muscular pump. Arteries are elastic tubes; unlike the rigid pipes of a water system they absorb the force of each heartbeat by expanding sideways to reduce the pressure of blood being delivered to distant parts of the system. Blood from a severed artery is bright scarlet and spurts in time with the heartbeat or pulse. Arteries have muscle and elastic tissue in their walls which, when injured, clamp down and draw back into the wound to stop bleeding. Arteries branch into arterioles and capillaries, the minute terminal vessels of the tree where gases are exchanged between blood and the tissue cells.

Venules collect blood from capillaries and empty into veins which return blood to the heart. Muscle exercise compresses the veins and pumps blood forward, aided by a series of one-way valves and a negative pressure vacuum in the chest that sucks venous blood back to the heart. Veins have little muscle or elastic tissue in their walls so do not retract on injury in the same way as arteries. Venous blood is darker red and wells up out of the wound.

The difference between arterial and venous bleeding is purely academic. All that is important is that bleeding must be stopped — and urgently.

SHOCK

Shock is how the body reacts to preserve life under threat.

Shock is a woolly term, blanketing a condition brought about by a reduction in the circulating blood volume for which there are many causes other than bleeding e.g. major burns, overwhelming infection, severe pain, heart failure.

In shock a chain of reactions develop. Bleeding reduces the amount of blood returning to the heart, which can consequently pump less blood into the circulation. The fall of blood pressure is registered in the main arteries leaving the heart by receptors which send nervous impulses to the brain. The pulse speeds up and pushes more blood per minute round the circulation in an attempt to correct the situation. Blood vessels in the extremities of the limbs clamp down and by-pass the skin, which becomes pale and cold; lack of oxygen makes the hands and feet waxy and blue. Several litres of blood from the periphery are pooled in the centre of the body where it is needed for the vital organs — brain, heart, lungs, and kidneys — which suffer damage quickly when deprived of oxygen.

If shock is not corrected the patient becomes breathless, thirsty and sick. Finally he is restless and confused, and unless the blood pressure is restored to normal by transfusion he will fall unconscious and may die.

Natural Halting of Bleeding.

a. Visible bleeding (from open wounds and in blood-soaked clothing).

i. Retraction. Muscular walls of vessels clamp down after injury to prevent further bleeding, and elastic tissue pulls the cut ends back into the wound.

ii. Clotting. After blood is shed it becomes solid clot, but this rarely happens within an intact vessel. Fibrin clot is formed by a complicated chain of chemical reactions involving the vessel wall itself, blood platelets, calcium, vitamin K, and prothrombin. These make thrombin which changes fibrinogen in the plasma into fibrin clot. Eventually fibrin hardens into fibrous healing tissue.

b. Hidden bleeding (in closed cavities like the chest or abdomen, and into loose tissue planes between muscles).

In a closed injury blood is unable to escape and tension builds up under the skin so the bleeding vessels are closed off by pressure, or continue to bleed into a cavity like the abdomen. Spilt red blood cells break down and release pigments which give the purple and yellow colour to a bruise. In massive closed bleeding the clotted blood partly liquifies; this causes pressure on neighbouring structures and may have to be evacuated to ease the pain.

Act.

A. Pressure.

i. Direct firm local pressure will stop most bleeding. Press steadily on a dressing of absorbent material placed well beyond the edges of the wound and be prepared to keep up the pressure for a long time. The dressing should preferably be sterile, (the inside of an ironed, folded handkerchief) but do not waste time looking; any reasonably clean material will do and someone else can worry about the infection later when you have saved the casualty from dying of loss of blood. Military 'wound

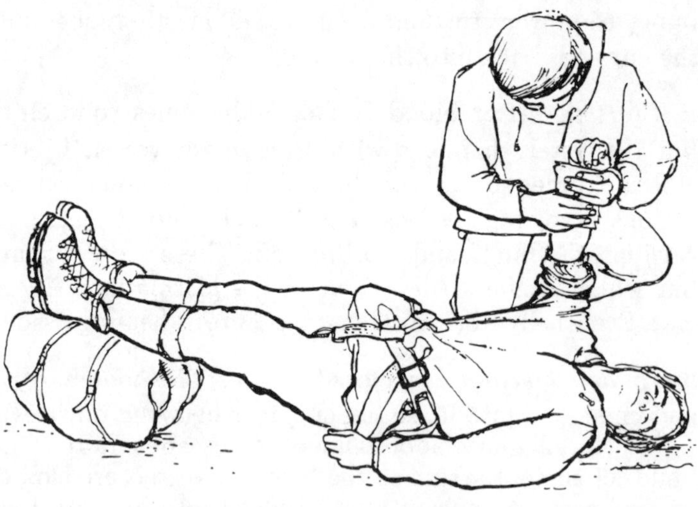

Figure 5.1 Pressure dressing for bleeding

dressings' are ideal; a compressed form of ladies' sanitary towel is as effective and far cheaper.

Do not remove the dressing when it becomes soaked, but pack more on top. Clot begins to form around the mesh of the fabric, and seals the bleeding ends of vessels and oozing capillaries. If you pull off the clot bleeding will start again. Cellulose gelatin mesh ('Oxycel', 'Gelfoam') dissolves in the wound and hastens clotting. Put an absorbent stretchy crepe bandage to keep the wound packing in place and to avoid movement that might restart bleeding.

ii. 'Pressure points' should be forgotten. They used to be taught to first-aiders, the principle being that if you press on the artery at the place where it passes over a bone lying near the surface, you can control the bleeding beyond. This may be useful for people with a working knowledge of anatomy but is impracticable in the situation of a climbing accident where much valuable time may be lost locating a pressure point and possibly not controlling the bleeding adequately while searching.

iii. Tourniquets can be dangerous so they should not be used. Bleeding from wounds can be adequately controlled by other methods. A tourniquet may obstruct veins without controlling arterial bleeding so the wound bleeds worse; it may be painful and cause restlessness; pressure may damage neighbouring structures such as nerves, and it may be forgotten and cause gangrene of the limb.

If ever a tourniquet has to be used because other methods have failed, always write a large T on the patient's forehead with a marker or lipstick, and write the time it was applied on a label tied round his neck.

iv. Clamps. On the rare occasion when a large artery is severed and bleeding cannot be controlled by pressure alone, it may be necessary to hold the ends with a surgical clamp (if available) and tie off the vessel with cotton.

B. Position.

i. Head down. If the patient is shocked and has a low blood pressure keep his head below the level of the body so his brain gets the benefit of gravity flow of blood. If blood pressure to the brain falls the casualty may become unconscious. The only exception to this is with head wounds when he should sit up.

ii. Feet up. Raise the feet by resting them on a rucksack; about 4 pints (2 litres) of blood, normally in the veins of the legs is pooled into the central circulation.

iii. Wounded part up. By elevating a wounded limb gravity lowers the arterial and venous pressure locally and allows clot to form.

C. Rest, reassurance, and pain relief.

i. Rest. Exercise speeds the heart to pump blood, and hence oxygen, faster to the muscles to produce energy; rest slows the heart and the blood flow. Resting the injured part encourages clotting and prevents the delicate web of early clot being broken or dislodged. Having dressed, packed and bandaged the wound, treat the part as though it were a fracture and splint it.

ii. Reassurance. Anxiety quickens the pulse and raises the blood pressure so, humane considerations apart, reassure the casualty that the bleeding has stopped and help will soon be at hand.

iii. Pain. People in pain, even if they are unconscious, become restless. Half measures are useless; severe pain in a fit adult can be treated with full doses of a drug like morphine (provided there is no difficulty with breathing or a head or chest injury). As well as relieving pain, these drugs give the casualty a pleasant feeling of warmth and well-being.

Pain relief can also be obtained from inhaling certain gases ('Entonox' which is a mixture of nitrous oxide, or 'laughing gas', and air). These are extremely safe and effective provided the patient holds the mask himself so it falls from his face if he has too much. Unfortunately the apparatus is bulky and heavy for use on mountain rescue, but is well worth the 15 lbs. weight if it is known that the casualty is in severe pain and will have to be carried far.

D. Further points:

i. Warmth. Excessive warming opens up the vessels of the skin and diverts blood from the central circulation where it is most needed. Someone shocked from blood loss feels cold because his skin vessels are constricted. It is unwise to reverse Nature's protection, for the casualty's apparent comfort. Nevertheless further loss of heat by exposure to the elements must be avoided.

ii. Fluids. If the casualty feels thirsty give him sips of water, enough to satisfy him without making him sick. After bleeding, body water is drawn into the blood by osmotic attraction to make up for lost plasma. Although not as good as replacing blood itself intravenously, fluid by mouth goes some way in helping redress the upset body water balance.

Look.

As soon as you have staunched severe bleeding, make written observations as a baseline to assess whether the casualty is improving or deteriorating. With hidden bleeding these may be your only guide.

1. Pulse. The pulse rate rises but the force felt on your fingers is weak because the blood pressure is low. This is only a rough guide.

2. Colour and temperature. The skin will be pale, and the hands and feet blue and cold. Pink colour returning to the face and warmth to the skin both show that vessels in the skin are open again and blood is being fully oxygenated.

3. Visible blood loss. From the amount of blood spilled you can estimate how serious the injury is and how much blood needs replacing. This information could be of vital importance to the doctors who are going to take over the casualty from you.

Blood is soaked up by clothing so an injury may appear small on the front of the casualty, but a pool of several pints may have formed below him on the stretcher. Turn him over and examine the clothing and blankets he is lying on.

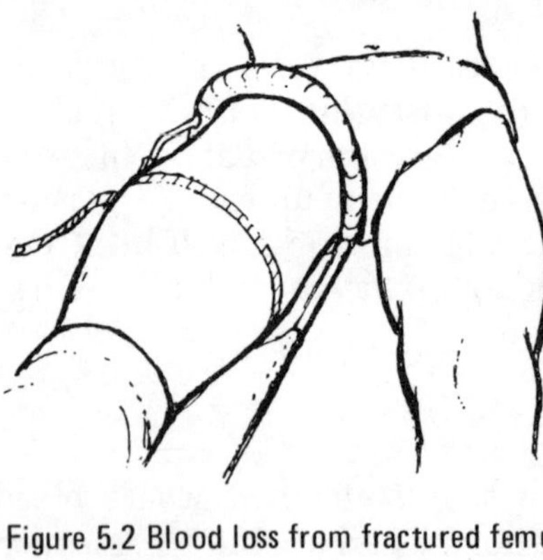

Figure 5.2 Blood loss from fractured femur

In closed wounds blood spreads along tissue planes causing swelling, or in cavities displacing the contents, the available space dictating the direction and pressure of the swelling. A fracture of the femur can bleed a litre into the thigh making it swell to twice its normal girth, but the swelling extends up to the hip and down to the knee.

Useful guidelines:—

— a person's hand is equivalent to about 1/10 of his blood volume, whether he is an adult or a child.

— an adult hand is roughly 1 pint ($\frac{1}{2}$ litre); push your fist into a pint beer glass to prove it.

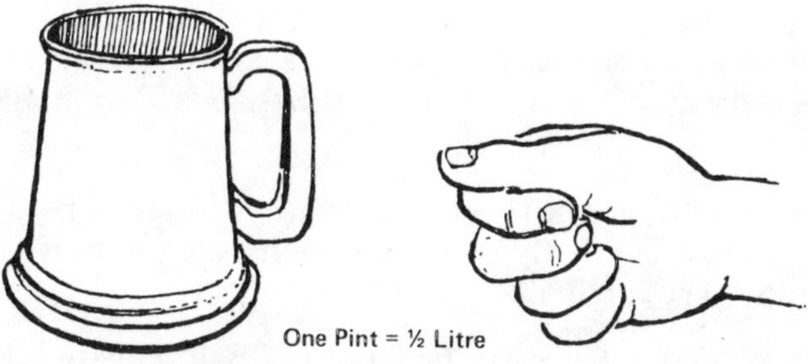

Figure 5.3 Estimation of blood loss

Blood Replacement.

Transfusion is the job of a doctor. You can however help by preparing the casualty on the mountain. Ask for his blood group; if he is unconscious look for a card in his wallet or a bracelet or medallion he may be wearing with all his relevant medical history imprinted on it. Send down any written information you can gather with the party going to seek help, who can pass it on to the hospital.

If there is a sterile needle and a syringe in your emergency kit and someone knows how to use them, take 10 ml. of blood from the patient's vein and either let it clot in the syringe or in a separate tube. The serum that settles out when the blood has clotted should be sent ahead with the rescue-seeking party. It can be used for preparing cross-matched blood for the casualty.

A transfusion can be set up at the site of an accident if a skilled person is in the rescue team. The arm should be splinted to prevent the needle moving as it may puncture the vein wall and the infusion will collect in the tissues causing a painful swelling. Even if blood is not available an intravenous infusion ('drip') set up on the spot has several advantages:—

— Any fluid will replace some of the depleted plasma volume and help to alleviate shock until blood is ready. A plasma substitute ('Dextran') is best but Normal Saline will do.

— Access to a vein is open as soon as blood is ready. If the victim suddenly collapses veins clamp down and may be very difficult to find.

— Intravenous drugs can be given in small repeated doses without the need to puncture the patient often. If he suddenly collapses this may be lifesaving.

Other Sources of Bleeding.

Climbers are most likely to encounter bleeding from wounds, but it is worth a quick look at other sorts of blood loss and the varied appearances of spilled blood. Always keep a specimen, however small, so it can be examined and analysed later in a laboratory. For the treatment of the conditions mentioned here, refer to the appropriate chapters later.

a. Saliva. A nosebleed, bitten tongue, bleeding gums or tooth socket, or injury to the nose, mouth or pharynx may lead to bright red blood trickling into the throat and being spat out mixed with saliva either as streaks or lumps of clot. A careful look with a strong light will usually reveal the source. One hidden and very serious cause may be a fracture of the base of the skull, when blood may also come from the ears.

b. Cough. Pink or rust-coloured flecks coughed up in frothy phlegm suggest that blood has come from the lungs, due possibly to pneumonia, pulmonary oedema or embolus (fluid or clot in the lungs).

c. Vomit. Swallowed blood irritates the stomach causing vomiting. If the blood has lain for any length of time in the stomach it becomes partly digested and changes colour from bright red to that of coffee grounds. Having excluded the causes in paragraph *a.*, bleeding peptic ulcer is most likely.

d. Urine. Blood may be so scanty as only to make the urine cloudy or slightly orange; if profuse it will be a deep red wine colour. When the story is of a blow in the loin, suspect bleeding from the kidney; if pain is acute and colicky a stone in the urinary passages is possible.

e. Stool. A little bright red blood streaked on the toilet paper suggests a crack at the anal margin from passing a constipated stool, or a small pile. Severe piles can bleed alarmingly, with clots. Digested blood from an ulcer that has passed the length of the gut produces a dark 'tarry' stool which can be confused with that of someone taking iron tablets.

f. Vagina. Normal menstrual calendars are often interrupted by a change in the pattern of living, particularly on climbing holidays. If there is any chance the woman may be pregnant consider the possibility that she is having an abortion (miscarriage).

6

Spinal Injury

Some spinal injuries are trivial, others are mortal or may become so if improperly handled. The aftermath of mismanagement will be serious even if the casualty survives.

How?

The spine consists of 24 vertebrae lying one on top of the other forming a supporting column between the skull and the pelvis. Forces are transmitted through the bony bodies of the vertebrae. The vertebral arches lie behind and form a tunnel in which the delicate spinal cord lies protected, and from which nerves leave and enter through side openings. Nerves for the arms leave highest, then those for the trunk, and lowest those for the legs.

Normally the spine can bend and twist around the many joints of the vertebrae. 'Discs' of semi-solid material lie between the vertebrae acting as washers that permit movement and take up forces of stress. They are held in place by ligaments and powerful overlying muscles running the entire length of the column.

A. Serious Injury

i. Fracture or dislocation (or both). The vertebrae are usually kept stable by the contraction of surrounding spinal muscles that ensure the integrity of the spinal canal, even if vertebrae are fractured. The fracture of a vertebra is much less important than the associated dam-

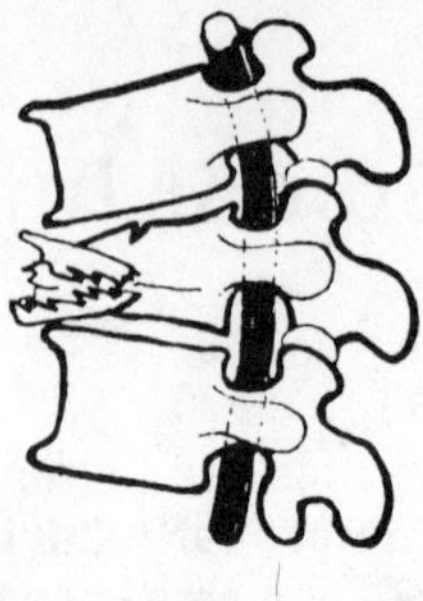

Figure 6.1a Crush fracture of vertebra – spinal cord unharmed

age to nerves that may be caused by vertebrae moving on each other; they may then sheer across the spinal cord, cutting nerve pathways and causing serious damage, or existing damage may be made worse.

The higher the spinal cord injury the more extensive will be the damage to nerve pathways below that level. If the cord is cut across in the neck, all four limbs, chest and abdomen will be paralysed; if the injury is in the middle of the back only the legs and bladder will be affected. Damage to the brain paralyses the opposite side

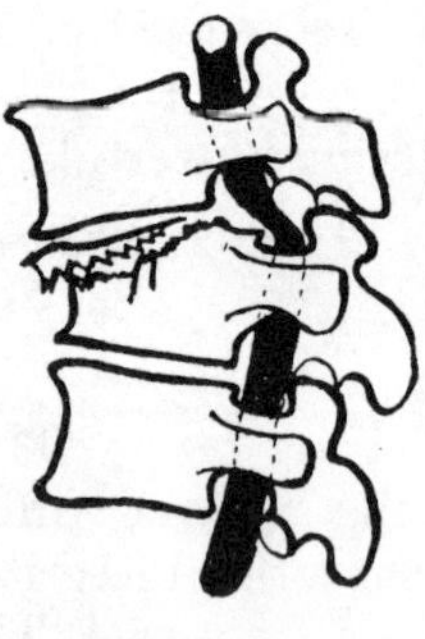

Figure 6.1b Spinal fracture – dislocation – spinal cord compressed

of the body because nerve pathways cross in the brain stem.

If a conscious patient complains of severe pain in his neck or back, even though he can move his limbs, treat him as if he has a fractured spine until proved otherwise. Unconscious patients usually respond to pain in the limbs. Care of the airway is still paramount as osbtruction will kill him.

a. Neck injury. This injury is potentially mortal. Handling a casualty clumsily may damage the spinal cord in the neck and paralyse breathing. Although the chest muscles are paralysed the diaphragm can usually maintain adequate breathing to keep the casualty alive. However, bruising and swelling may spread upwards in the spinal cord affecting the phrenic nerve to the diaphragm. Unless mechanical breathing is available the casualty will die, since you will not be able to keep up assisted breathing for long enough.

To make an accurate diagnosis on the mountainside is difficult. So move the casualty with all speed and without further damage to a hospital where he can be X-rayed and given expert treatment.

Suspect a fractured neck if:—

a. the climber has fallen from a height and injured his head.

b. he complains of pain in his neck or holds his neck in an abnormal position. Look for bruising or abrasion of the skin of his neck.

c. he complains of loss of feeling, or tingling and numbness in the hands or arms.

d. a gap can be felt in the equal spacing of the prominences of the vertebrae when you run your fingers along the spine. This sign is not as obvious in fractures of the neck as in those of the back.

b. Back injury. Though unlikely to kill the climber outright a back injury may paralyse him from the waist down. He may be surprisingly tranquil and say he feels as if he has been cut in half with no feeling below the waist. At the site of injury he will feel pain, which radiates round his middle from that level and shoots down his legs. If he can move his fingers and toes and if he can feel light touch on his skin you may be sure he has no nerve damage; but do not move his limbs actively yourself or you may cause further injury.

Act.

Do the best you can; if the spine is fractured and/or dislocated the injury will be so great you are unlikely to worsen the damage, but by not moving the patient he may die from other causes. The ideal situation described in text-books very rarely obtains when you are out on a mountain. The climber with a suspected fracture of the spine may have to be moved to a safer position in order to resuscitate him, or have to be lifted onto a stretcher.

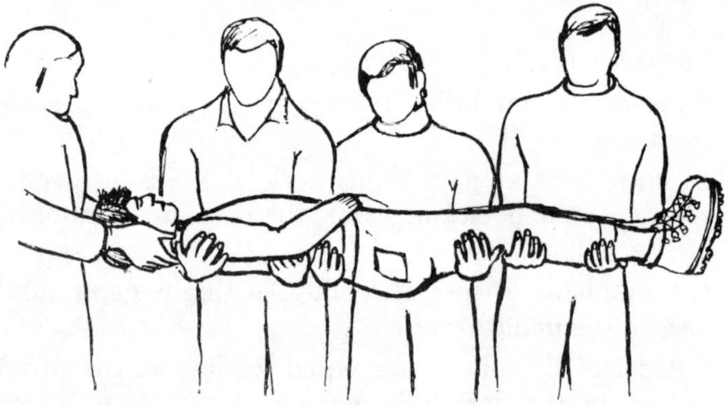

Figure 6.2 Carrying a spinal fracture 'in one piece'

Move him 'in one piece' to avoid increasing the displacement of any vertebrae which may be dislocated. One person holds the head, one the legs and another two the body, and all the rescuers work together so the casualty's head does not twist on his shoulders nor his body on his pelvis.

Comfort.

Relieve pain with full doses of analgesic drugs, but if the chest muscles are affected beware of morphine because it depresses breathing.

Carry.

a. Neck injury. Lay the casualty flat on a stretcher. Do not try to correct any deformity of his head or neck. Splint his neck with two rolls of clothing on either side of his head or a pair of boots, soles outwards, uppers under the neck, held in position by a bandage round his forehead. A collar can be

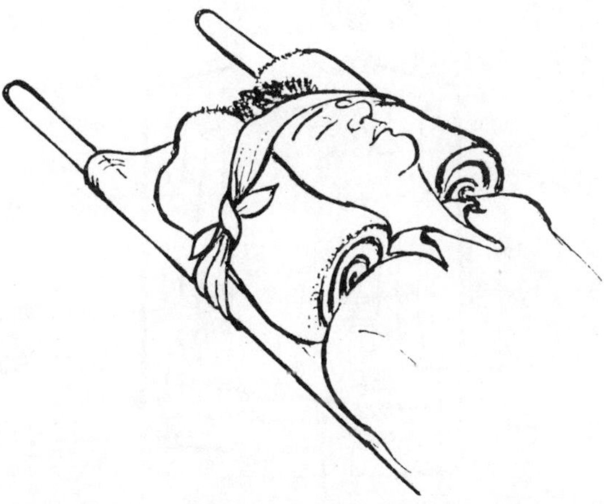

Figure 6.3 Neck splint

made of cardboard or rolled newspaper wrapped in clothing.

Tie the injured climber firmly to the stretcher so his body cannot move on his splinted head. A 'spinal board' is a useful piece of equipment to be carried by rescue teams.

b. Back injury. If the patient is conscious and in full control of his airway he will probably be most comfortable lying on his back on a stretcher. If he is unconscious, the draining position is not feasible as he will roll around. So lay him face down with his head turned to the side; his spine will be slightly bowed and less likely to dislocate further, but avoid any twisting movement. Pad between his knees and ankles to prevent points of pressure, and bandage his legs together with a figure-of-eight so he may be more easily moved 'in one piece'.

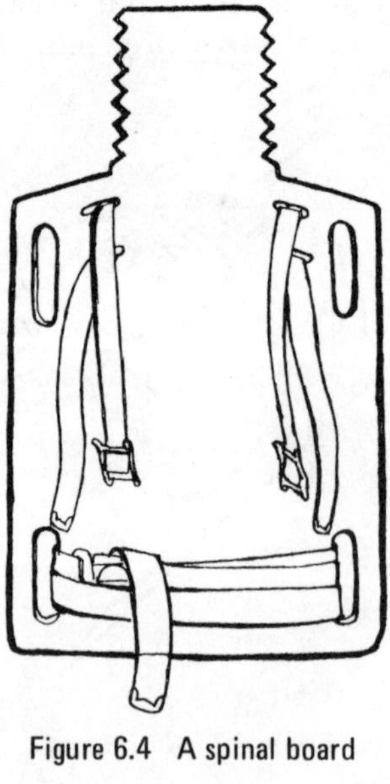

Figure 6.4 A spinal board

Care of Paralysed Persons

Paralysed persons are liable to damage themselves because they cannot feel pain and the normal sensations of touch, pressure and temperature. When asleep we unconsciously shift our position every few minutes to distribute the weight of our body evenly over the surface on which we are lying. A paralysed person lies still, and unrelieved pressure on the skin cuts off the blood supply locally causing painless sores which may pass unnoticed.

Nursing

Careful nursing is needed to protect the patient from injuring himself. Pressure sores can develop in a few hours and take weeks to heal. Nurse the casualty on a firm surface with no wrinkled bedding, clothes or objects in his pockets on which he may lie and so cause pressure. Pad bony prominences and body hollows, especially behind the neck, and loosen tight clothing. Turn him every two hours to encourage blood to return to areas that have been pressed on. If he has lost control of his bladder or bowels keep him clean and dry. Other complications that threaten the paralysed person are infection of the lungs (pneumonia) and of the kidneys (pyelitis).

B. Less Serious Back Injuries

Though not mortal these are included here for comparison with severe spinal injuries.

i. Back strain ('Lumbago'). Abnormal stresses which pull or tear the ligaments can bruise or strain the back. In order to protect the vertebral joint the spinal muscles go into spasm, causing pain.

Act.

Rest, local heat, avoiding the precipitating cause, and allowing Nature time to heal, is usually enough to cure lumbago.

ii. Slipped disc ('Sciatica'). If a disc prolapses through a gap in the spinal ligaments, which usually happens posteriorly at their weakest point, it may press on the spinal nerve roots causing pain and tingling down the distribution of the nerve – the arms if a cervical (neck) vertebra, the legs if a lumbar (low back) vertebra. Sciatica is the pain felt in the leg down the course of the sciatic nerve, which is commonly pressed on by a prolapsed disc in the lumbar region. If pressure is not released the nerve may be permanently damaged with loss of sensation and muscle power, and cause severe pain.

Act.

Treat the pain and evacuate the patient speedily.

7

Chest Injury

In a serious climbing accident both the head and chest may be injured but the chest can pass unnoticed because of the more obvious head injury. So head *and* chest must be examined as injuries to either may be mortal.

The chest may be *crushed* by tumbling onto rock, by a falling stone or by sudden tightening of a climbing rope or harness after a fall (closed injury), or it may be *punctured* by a spike of rock or the pick of an ice-axe (open injury).

The casualty may show few signs of injury. His colour will be difficult to see if the light is poor or if he is unwashed and weather-beaten; his breathing pattern may be obscured by his clothing. But a climber can die more quickly from a chest injury than from a head injury, abdominal injury or fractured bones. So in the first rapid look over the victim have a good light handy. Open his clothing so you can see the whole chest and not just inside the top shirt button; as most quiet breathing is done with the lower chest or upper abdomen, you may easily not notice it.

How?

i) Structure

The chest is an expanding cage that houses the lungs which branch repeatedly into finer and finer passages (bronchi, bronchioles), and end in millions of air sacs (alveoli).

The chest acts as a bellows with the lungs suspended inside the cavity. It expands by the ribs moving upwards and outwards, rotating like the handle of a bucket round two fixed points fore and aft where they are attached to

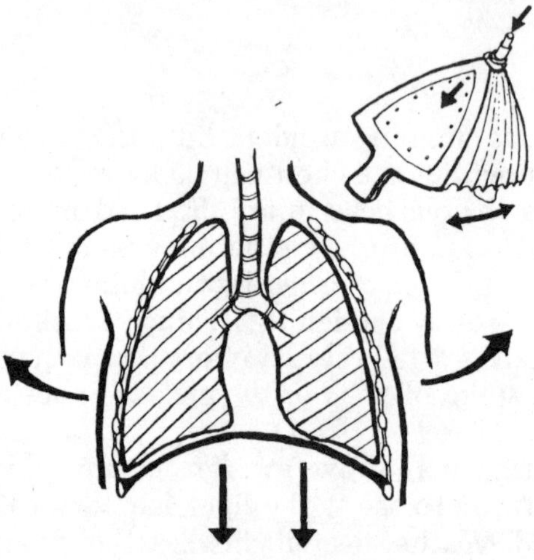

Figure 7.1a Inspiration

the vertebral column behind and the sternum (breast bone) in front. At the same time the diaphragm, a dome shaped muscular sheet separating the chest from the abdomen, moves downwards like a piston increasing the vertical diameter of the chest and creating a vacuum or negative pressure within the chest. Other accessory muscles in the neck which are not normally used can also assist breathing. The inside of the chest and the outside of the lung are covered with a very fine slippery surface, the pleura, that allows one surface to glide across the other without friction. The two are normally closely opposed with an unmeasurable space between. A low vacuum in this pleural space holds the lung expanded against the chest wall, resisting the natural retractile force of its elastic fibres, which are responsible for expiration. If this vacuum is destroyed by letting air into the pleural space there is nothing to hold the lung open

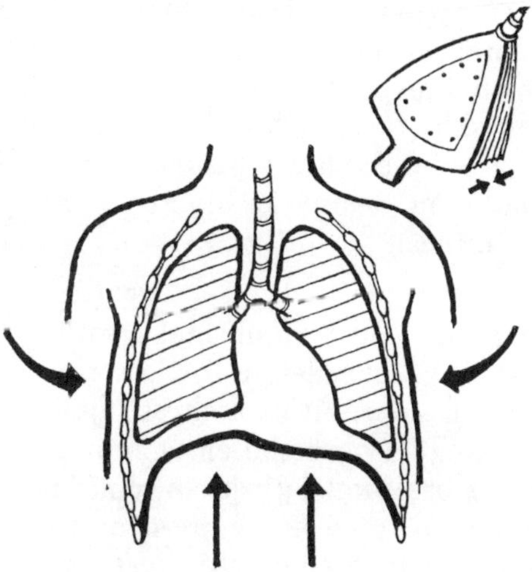

Figure 7.1b Expiration

and it collapses (pneumothorax). However, when filled with air on taking a breath, the lungs stretch like a blown-up balloon.

ii) Normal Breathing. (Function)

The lungs fill with air on inspiration. Oxygen passes into the blood across the walls of the lung alveoli, which are but a single cell thick, so gases can be exchanged to and fro between air in the alveoli and blood in the capillaries of the lung circulation.

Carbon dioxide passes in the reverse direction and in expiration it is discharged from the lungs to the outside air.

General Management of a Chest Injury

Look.

a. At the patient's face. If oxygen fails to reach the blood, either owing to airway block or a disordered chest, the blood changes colour from bright red to purple. Together with the pallor induced by the shock of the accident the skin turns a bluish cyanotic colour most clearly seen around the lips especially on the shiny inner mucous membrane. Search for blood-stained spittle coming from the mouth.

b. At the patient's chest. In normal breathing both sides of the chest have a quiet, effortless rhythm and rise equally on both sides. After a chest injury breathing is shallow and irregular and the chest moves unequally. A skin wound or bruising suggests mischief below the surface which is confirmed if the chest on the injured side does not move. Quite adequate breathing can be done by the diaphragm alone with barely any chest movement so look at the upper abdomen for breathing movements. When breathing is under stress accessory muscles are brought into action to help; with each breath the nostrils flare, the neck muscles tighten and the muscles in the spaces between the ribs are indrawn.

The chest may be sucked in during inspiration instead of expanding, which is called paradoxical breathing (see later).

Listen.

— for the croaking sound of obstructed breathing

— for a hiss of air escaping from, or a sucking noise of air entering, a chest wound.

Feel.

— the rib cage gently for tenderness and for an unstable segment of the chest wall.

— for chest movement by lightly placing the palms of your hands flat on the front and side of the bare chest and notice them being moved apart with each breath.

— with the flat of the hand laid over the chest for crackling, like the rustle of brown paper being folded, which suggests escaped gas in the tissues.

Act. . . Immediately

— clear the airway (see Chapter 2). This is vital and urgent.

— place a clean dressing over any wound and seal it with strapping tape to prevent the escape or entry of air.

— turn the casualty so he is lying on the *injured* side of his chest.

This simple action makes sure that:

— he is in the draining position, thus keeping the airway clear of blood and secretions.

— any moving segments of the chest wall or broken ribs are splinted by the weight of his own body making the chest cage stable and rigid.

— a penetrating wound remains sealed by the gravity pressure of the weight of the body.

— encourage coughing to remove blood or secretions from the air passages.

— if cyanosis persists despite the above — give oxygen (if available) — consider tracheotomy (doctor).

Specific Chest Injuries

A. Lung Injury

1. Pneumothorax. Air may enter the pleural space from outside of the chest by way of a penetrating wound, or from within because of a burst alveolus or bronchus, or rupture of the oesophagus. The vacuum that normally exists in the pleural space is destroyed so the lung collapses and the chest cavity fills with air. If the wound seals itself, air in the chest may absorb slowly and the lung re-expand; this can be speeded by inserting a needle and drawing off the air. However, if the penetrating wound remains 'open' with connection to the outside, air is sucked in and out of the chest through the wound instead of through the mouth into the lungs. Until the wound is sealed and the vacuum restored the lung will not be able to function.

Act.

If breathing becomes embarrassed from air or blood or both within the chest, and especially if pressure rises, decompression is urgent. Push a wide-bore needle into the space between the second and third ribs just below the middle of the clavicle and cover the end with a finger, removing it to allow a hiss of air to escape on expiration; then replace the finger to seal the needle when he breathes in. When all the air appears to have been removed and his breathing is easier, pull the needle out and cover the tiny hole with a plaster. Air decompression may have to be repeated if the chest fills up again.

2. Haemothorax. Bleeding into the chest cavity from a wound of the lung or injured blood vessels can pool blood in the pleural space and collapse the lung in the same way as a pneumothorax, but it is more serious as the bleeding

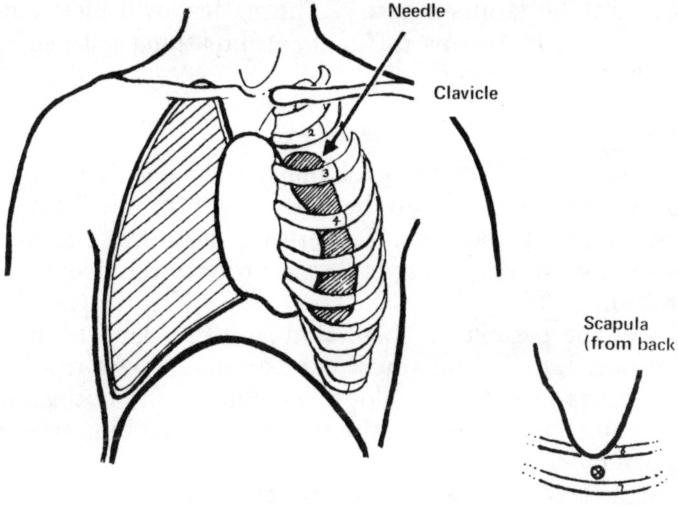

Figure 7.2 Pneumothorax — needling

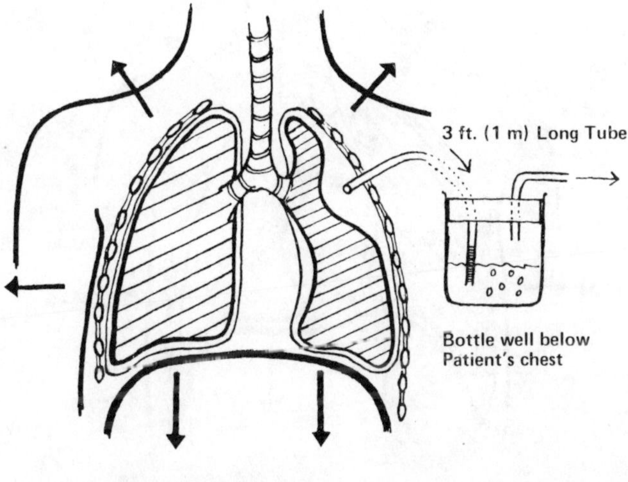

Figure 7.3 Pneumothorax — underwater-seal drain

may not be stopped easily. The patient will have continued and increasing difficulty in breathing with signs of shock from blood loss.

Act.

If bleeding is the main problem put the needle into the lower part of the chest between the 6th and 7th ribs just below the scapula. 'Underwater-seal' drainage may be necessary using a large tube, in order to remove blood and fluid.

Get the patient to hospital quickly. Transport him in the position he finds most comfortable. There is some advantage in sitting as blood can sink to the bottom of the chest and air rise to the top, leaving the lung free to expand.

If, despite all these measures, the patient's breathing is inadequate you will have to consider tracheostomy

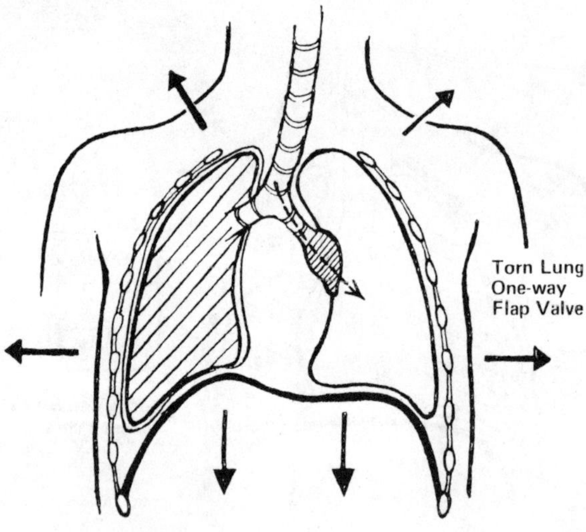

Figure 7.4 Tension pneumothorax

(q.v. p. 17) weighing the difficulty of doing this as an emergency procedure against the danger of the patient dying from suffocation.

3. Tension pneumothorax (sucking wound of the chest). If the chest or lung wound does not seal, a flap of tissue may act as a one-way valve so air is sucked in with each breath but the flap-valve is closed on expiration. The chest fills with more air each breath; the air has no means of escape and the pressure can rise so high that the mediastinum (trachea, heart and great arteries and veins) is pushed across to the opposite side. The patient becomes severely short of oxygen, goes blue, and his heart may stop. Urgent, on-the-spot action is mandatory.

Act.

Seal the hole immediately with a sterile gauze dressing. Greasy tulle-gras clings to the edges of the wound making it air-tight. Strap or bandage a thick dressing of gauze or

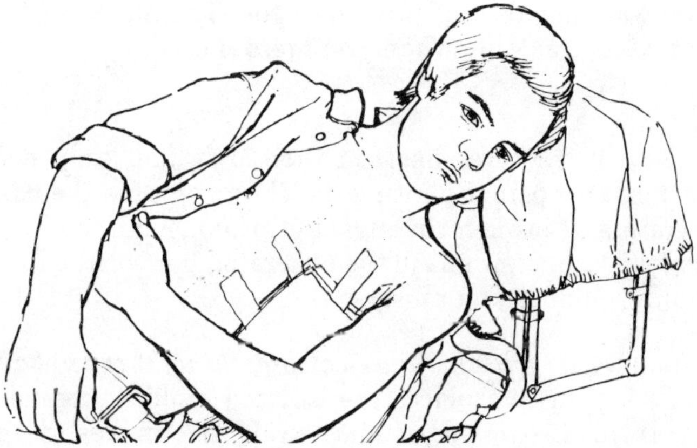

Figure 7.5 Chest dressing

cotton-wool in place and lay the patient on his injured side so that the pressure of his body weight holds the dressing in place.

Air can be removed from the pneumothorax as described above.

B. Rib Cage Injury

1. Fractured ribs. A simple rib fracture does not jeopardise the stability of the chest wall; it is painful but not serious. The pain is due to broken ends of the bone grating against sensitive periosteum, the tissue that covers all bones and is well supplied with pain nerves.

When a number of ribs are fractured the chest wall may be indented and the jagged rib ends puncture the underlying lung releasing air into the pleura (pneumothorax) or tear the intercostal vessels causing a pool of blood in the chest (haemothorax). Breathing is shallow and coughing feeble because of the pain, so secretions pool at the bases of the lungs and if not removed will lead to pneumonia later. If the pleura lining the chest wall is breached, air may leak into the tissues of the chest wall and rise up into the neck. The bubbles of air can be felt crackling when you press the skin.

Act.

Simple rib fractures heal on their own and only need treatment for pain. Splinting the chest prevents the painful grating of broken rib ends, but prolonged immobility may lead to pneumonia in the unaerated part of the lung. So only splint if you must.

2. 'Flail' chest with paradoxical breathing. If several ribs are broken in two places the isolated middle fragments may form a segment of chest wall that moves in the opposite direction to the rest of the chest during breathing. It is sucked in on inspiration when the chest nor-

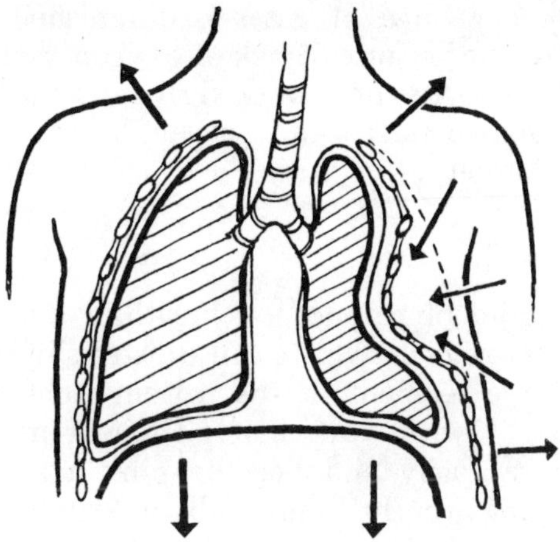

Figure 7.6 "Flail" chest – paradoxical breathing

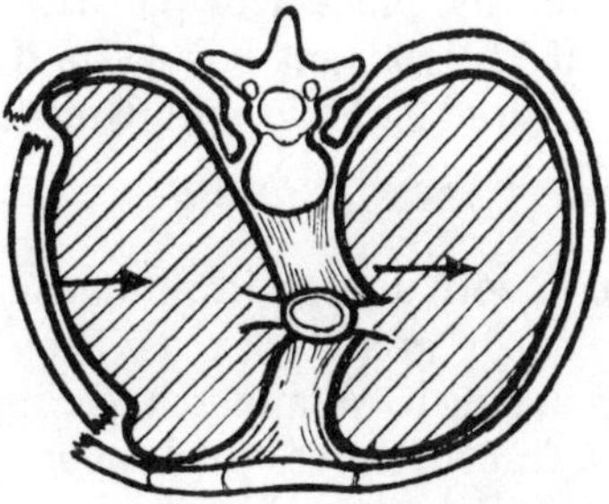

Figure 7.7 "Flail" chest – paradoxical breathing

mally expands, and is blown out on expiration when the chest deflates. This is called paradoxical breathing. All the effort of breathing is spent in moving the unsupported 'flail' segment rather than in shifting air in and out of the lungs, which become poorly ventilated. The result is that the exchange of gases is diminished and the patient goes blue because of lack of oxygen. Extra efforts to breathe increase the paradoxical movement making the situation worse, so the patient becomes anxious, restless and sweaty.

Act.

A small amount of paradoxical breathing may need no treatment. If severe enough to cause distress in breathing, fix the mobile segment of the patient's chest wall by pressing on it with your hand. He will immediately breathe more easily and become pink again. Strap a wound dressing over the injured ribs and turn the patient on that side in order to prevent the segment of chest wall moving in and out.

i. Splinting. Bind the arm, bent at the elbow, across the chest. Clothing left in place will pad the chest and give added support. If the patient has to lie down make him turn onto the injured side so splinting the broken ribs under the weight of his body.

ii. Pain. Treat pain with analgesics, but use morphine and pethidine only with great care as they both depress breathing. Long-acting local anaesthetic injected directly into the site of a fracture gives prolonged pain relief, but beware of slipping between the ribs and puncturing the lung.

iii. Breathing. Encourage deep breathing and coughing to clear the lung of secretions. Infection is a likely sequel to chest injury especially if there is blood in the chest to act as a medium for bacteria to grow in. If the patient has a fever, or if he coughs up thick yellow or green spittle give a broad-spectrum antibiotic.

iv. Surgical correction. This is only necessary if paradoxical movement embarrasses breathing and other measures fail. In desperation you can pass a wire round the ribs and pull outwards on the fragment. In hospital the patient would be put on a mechanical ventilator.

3. Chest wall injury. The skin and muscles overlying the injury may be severely bruised with as much as two pints of blood hidden in the bruise.

8

Exposure

The Shorter Oxford English Dictionary defines the verb 'expose' as, '. . to leave without shelter or defence; to imperil'. Exposure is a useful word for climbers to describe a complex group of conditions and body reactions that scientists more accurately call Mountain Hypothermia. Other factors besides climatic cold contribute to exposure, especially fatigue, anxiety and injury.

Exposure occurs as readily on the British hills as in the high Himalaya because wet cold is more chilling than dry cold. Good planning and preparation for every expedition, however short, will reduce the chances of exposure, careful observation can detect it early and prompt action will avert disaster. Eric Langmuir says in his book 'Mountain Leadership', "There is some danger that our attention may be diverted from the bread and butter business of prevention by the spectacular recommendations on the treatment of exposure cases. Many long-cherished cures have been thrown out of the window along with St. Bernard dogs, brandy and hot water bottles. Think ahead. There is no substitute for careful planning."

Wet cold is a dangerous enemy and the killer of the unprepared.

Plan the day's march so it is well within the limits of the party and geared to the ability of the weakest member. The distance you can cover and your speed will vary with the loads carried, the type of terrain and the weather. The person most likely to suffer from exposure is one who has walked too far too fast, carried too heavy a load and is hungry, demoralized and exhausted. If the weather changes, be prepared to abandon the original plan and take an easier or shorter route off the mountain.

Children and adolescents withstand cold less well than adults because they have a large surface area in proportion to their weight, and generally carry less subcutaneous fat. Children do not have the experience or training that build up reserves of stamina and mental fibre. They become demoralized, give up hope and flag early unless they have a strong and encouraging leader.

HOW?

Temperature Control

The temperature of the central body core is kept close to normal 37°C by our own delicate 'thermostat' that balances heat gain and heat loss. The body has a central 'core' which must be kept at a constant temperature in order that the vital organs it contains — brain, heart, liver, kidneys, — may function at their most efficient level. Most heat exchange takes place in the surrounding 'shell' of skin, subcutaneous fat and muscle which is cooler than the core (about 33°C).

A rise or fall in temperature of one degree brings on noticeable symptoms and if the temperature of the central body core drops a few degrees a person may die. Body temperature is usually measured by a thermometer placed under the tongue, which is 1°C below the core temperature. In an unconscious person breathing through his mouth, this may be difficult, but the alternative method of using a thermometer placed in the rectum is impracticable on a mountainside. The armpit is not accurate enough. A special low-reading thermometer is needed to register below 35°C.

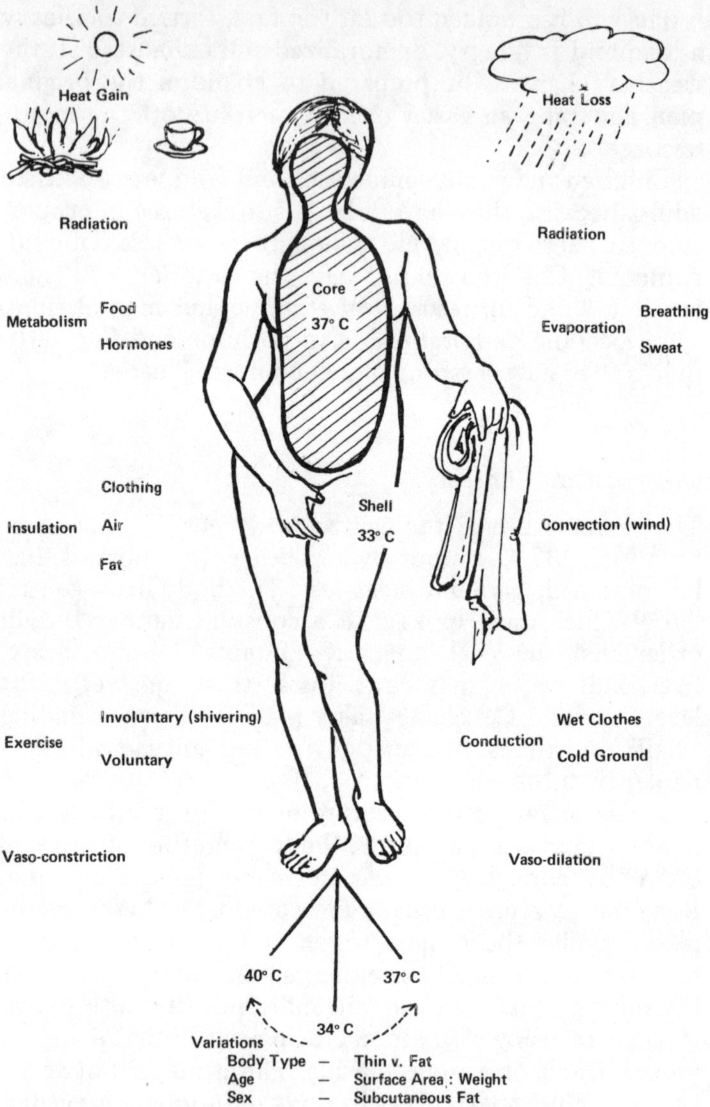

Figure 8.1 Body temperature

The body thermostat is like a pair of scales that must be kept in balance. If the scales tip we take conscious steps to correct the situation by either gaining or losing heat. But if heat continues to be lost despite all attempts to conserve it, for example, lying wet on a mountain in a cold wind, the body core temperature may fall to a seriously low level.

A. Body Heat is *Lost* by:

i. Wind (convection). At any steady temperature, wind speed determines the chill you feel; air temperature alone is meaningless as a measure of cold. On a windless sunny day with the temperature at 40° below zero Centigrade you can walk about in shirtsleeves, but the least puff of wind will send you hurrying for your warm clothing.

The graph shows the chilling effect of various combinations of wind speed and temperature, a measure referred to as the 'wind-chill index'. Wind chills by lowering the outside air temperature, destroying air insulation and by using up energy in withstanding its force.

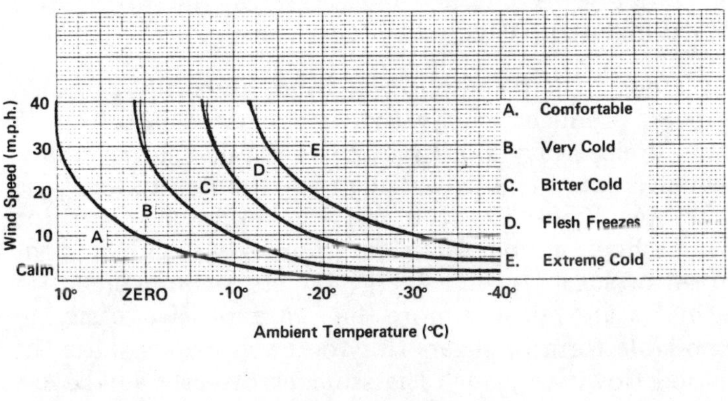

Figure 8.2 Wind-chill chart

ii. Conduction. Heat flows directly from the warm body to wet clothes and cold objects, like the ground on which you may be sitting.

iii. Evaporation.

Sweating. Loss of heat by evaporation of sweat lowers the temperature. One pint ($\frac{1}{2}$ litre) of fluid a day is lost through the skin, but in hot climates or after heavy exercise this loss may be far greater.

Breathing. Warm breath condenses in cold air, and breathing cold air cools the blood in the lungs. Animals that do not sweat, pant to lose heat through rapid breathing instead.

iv. Blood vessel dilatation. Shock caused by injury complicates exposure. Cold causes blood vessels to constrict, but this control fails in shock and the vessels dilate and lose heat to the outside air.

B. Body Heat is *Gained* by:

i. Radiation. Sun and fire give off heat.

ii. Exercise. Voluntary muscle work and involuntary shivering use up energy to produce heat.

iii. Food. The metabolism of food, especially carbohydrates, produces energy that is converted into heat. A man doing heavy work requires 4–4,500 calories a day, which is equivalent to walking twelve miles (20 km.) and climbing 2,500 ft. (750 m.) e.g. round the Snowdon Horseshoe. Carbohydrate is most quickly absorbed in the form of sugar. Instant energy tablets recommended for athletes are nothing more than an expensive, easily assimilable form of sugar. Hot food and drinks warm the blood flowing through the stomach directly and have a great morale-boosting effect.

C. Body Heat is *Stored* by:

i. Insulation. Air and fat retain heat as they are poor conductors and therefore good insulators; water is a good conductor allowing heat to drain away. Animals raise the hairs of their fur to trap air in the same way as we get goose-pimples when we are cold. Shetland wool, feathers of eider or duck-down, string vests and cellular materials insulate by trapping a layer of air in the interstices of the fabric.

Finely woven fabric is windproof and prevents draughts from displacing the warm air by convection. Clothing saturated with water loses 90% of its insulation against wind and cold because wet clothes cling to the skin destroying the layer of air, and also heat is absorbed into the water by conduction. So clothing must be both waterproof and windproof. Waterproof material is also windproof but it needs some ventilation to reduce the condensation on the inside of the garment, that can make you as wet as if it is raining outside.

Wool retains warmth even when wet; its cellular structure does not collapse as duck-down does, and it still provides effective insulation by trapping air. The early Everesters managed to climb to 28,000 ft. in Norfolk jackets dipped in a solution of alum to repel water, six layers of Shetland wool pullovers and long woollen stockings. Tweed breeches do not absorb water as do cotton jeans which give poor protection to the legs, an area from which much heat can be lost.

Parts of the body exposed to the elements must be covered since blood flowing near the surface is liable to cooling. Half the body's heat production can be lost from an uncovered head; a balaclava helmet allows a minimum area of the head to be exposed to the air. Remember, when your feet are cold, put on your hat. The old-fashioned red flannel kidney-warmer serves a real purpose in keeping draughts away from the mid-riff.

Clothing should fit closely round the neck, wrists and ankles to prevent draughts and keep out water. A towelling or wool scarf, buttons or elastic at the wrists, and inner trousers tucked into the socks all help to this end, but they must not be so tight as to constrict the flow of blood. Hence mittens are preferable to gloves because they allow free movement of the fingers which warm each other by their proximity. Outer trousers can be left out so air can circulate under them and rain runs over the tops of the boots.

ii. Blood vessel clamp-down (vaso-constriction). Vessels in the shell clamp down in order to pool warm blood in the central core and prevent heat loss to the cold outside air by convection. Smooth muscle in the walls of the blood vessels is under automatic reflex control.

Be vigilant to detect exposure early and to stop it worsening. A multitude of vague signs may be the only warning you will get. Once exposed, a climber deteriorates quickly and unless treated he may die. Signs develop as the body temperature falls, but they may not necessarily occur in the order given below.

— Mild exposure. 37°–33°C

The casualty complains of feeling cold and of cramps in his muscles. The only sign of exposure may be his uncharacteristic behaviour. This may be difficult to detect unless someone knows his normal personality and performance. He may be excited and swearing, or lethargic with unusually slow actions. His skin will be cold, pale and bluish. As he gets colder his normal shivering becomes quite uncontrollable, he is unco-ordinated with slurred speech and visual disturbances and he stumbles, trips and falls.

— Serious exposure. Below 32°C

Shivering stops so the casualty's main self-protective mechanism has gone. His muscles become stiff and rigid and his breathing quickens. He behaves irrationally, so he may be violent and aggressive or quite apathetic. Finally he has convulsions and slips into coma. Irregular heart beats herald the onset of fibrillation of the heart ventricles which will be the ultimate cause of his death.

Act.

The aim of treating a person suffering from exposure is to prevent further loss of heat and to restore his body temperature to normal.

A. On the Mountain

— Mild exposure. It is very difficult to decide whether to try to get down off the mountain and out of the conditions that are causing the illness, or whether to stay put in adverse circumstances and to call out a rescue party, which may take several hours to arrive.

If you decide that the climber is fit to go on, first take a rest. Shelter out of the wind, have something to eat and, if possible, make a hot drink. This may give a tired person the impetus to walk off the hillside unaided before he becomes a victim of serious exposure, when he will certainly need a stretcher. Alcohol is traditionally banned for anyone suffering from exposure because, in theory, the drug dilates blood vessels and heat is lost thereby. A person has to be paralytically drunk before he loses a significant amount of heat, but the nip of brandy may do wonders for his spirits. The danger of alcohol is that it can cause a sudden fall in blood sugar because it depresses the mobilization of fuel reserves which go to make glucose. This causes temperature regulation to fail, especially after heavy exercise. So always hand out sweets before passing round the hip-flask, and do not let them swig the lot.

Descend at the pace of the casualty to a camp or hut where he can be thoroughly warmed.

– Serious exposure. Stop and put the victim in a 'Poly-bag', a strong polythene bag (120 gauge minimum) 7 ft. (2.2 m.) long and 3 ft. (1 m.) wide, roomy enough to take a fully clothed man. He should be wrapped in all the spare clothing; a duvet jacket or a sleeping bag carried in a rucksack in case of such an emergency may be life-saving. Every large party is wise to carry a lightweight bivouac or 'tunnel' tent that is erected over aluminium or bamboo hoops. If you do not have a tent build a windproof and waterproof shelter, but while you are doing this insulate the casualty from the cold ground below him with clothes, rucksacks or bracken.

Calculate your position on the map accurately and write down the map reference together with a message about the condition of the casualty (see page 212). Send the strongest and most competent member of the party for help, having agreed with him a signal to show your position to the returning rescue party.

If you can move the victim into a tent, change his wet clothes for dry ones, but this may be impossible in the open air. Put him in a sleeping bag with anything available to heat him such as hot water in a metal water-bottle or heated stones, wrapped in a cloth to prevent him being burnt. Try to get him to take a hot drink. A small cooker or self-heating soup cans make a drink that will provide a big boost to morale even if it does not significantly raise the body temperature. A group huddled together inside a tent with a stove burning will generate a lot of heat. Do not forget the other members of the party who may also be very cold and will need sustenance for the long hard job of rescue. Reassurance and strong leadership raise wilting spirits.

If the exposed climber improves he should be encouraged to walk down on his own towards the direction of the rescue party as the exercise will warm him. If you can avoid a stretcher evacuation you will save a lot of hard and dangerous work during which the victim will become even colder from lying immobile and rescuers lives are in danger. This twilight decision time demands much courage.

B. At Base

If the casualty is very cold rewarm him rapidly in a bath of water at about 44°C. A water thermometer and a low-reading thermometer are useful pieces of equipment to have in a base medical pack. In emergency remember the old aphorism, 'If you put your baby in the bath and it goes pink, then the water's too hot for your elbow'. Water that feels comfortably warm to the touch is about 44°C.

Place him in the bath fully clothed because very cold people curl up in a ball and removing their clothes is almost impossible. His cold wet clothes will drop the temperature of the bath which will need adjusting rapidly. You can strip him later when he relaxes as he warms up with his trunk and neck submerged and his limbs outside, since your prime aim is to raise the core temperature and not to worry about the shell. As blood from the cold limbs returns to the centre it will cool the rewarmed blood, ('after-drop') so it is necessary to keep the temperature of the water bath up by repeatedly topping up with hot water and stirring all the time to prevent scalding the patient.

As he warms up he may start to shiver violently and painfully, and he will need analgesic drugs. When he is fully rewarmed remove him from the bath and put him, head-downhill, into a bed that has been heated with hot-water-bottles in a room that can be kept hot. Watch carefully as he can collapse from 'after-drop' owing to cold blood returning to the core from the shell that has not been completely rewarmed.

If he is unconscious it is not safe to use a bath. An alternative is to place his hands in very warm water, though this is very slow. The rhythm of the heart can become disturbed in hypothermia. Flutter of the auricles, felt at the pulse, is alarming but in fact needs no treatment; fibrillation of the ventricles signifies impending doom. Both the diagnosis and the special equipment needed to restore normal rhythm are beyond the scope of the mountain rescuer and can only be done in hospital. So if this happens just pray hard.

Breathing warm humidified air transfers heat rapidly and directly to the heart and the lung circulation. This raises the temperature of the core albeit not as quickly as by immersion. A method has recently been described whereby a casualty breathes oxygen, from a small portable cylinder, that passes through a canister of soda-lime. The carbon dioxide from his exhaled breath reacts with the soda-lime, generating heat and moisture.

This method has the advantage over immersion that it is without danger of 'after-drop' and of lethal heart irregularities, it prevents further loss of heat from the expired air, and the apparatus can be carried by a rescue party, and rewarming can be started on the mountain. It should be emphasized that it is not a substitute for, but an adjunct to, conventional hot bath re-warming.

At extremely low temperatures the body may go into a state of 'suspended animation' as hibernating animals do. The oxygen requirements of the brain and heart are less, a fact used in the principle of super-cooling during open heart surgery to allow the surgeon longer to operate on the heart than the usual allowable stoppage time of four minutes. Breathing and heartbeat slow down greatly, but they may be normal for that particular degree of hypothermia.

Even if you think the person is dead, try to rewarm him. Only diagnose death if you fail to revive him by adequate rewarming. A severely exposed person, who is still alive, may have no shivering reflex, stiff muscles like rigor mortis, pale bloodless skin and barely perceptible heartbeat and breathing. The only sure sign of death is when the pupils of the eyes are large and do not react by becoming constricted to a small aperture when a light is shone into them.

So do not give up easily; he may be alive yet. 'Corpses' have been known to wake up in a nice warm mortuary.

9

Abdominal Injury

Serious abdominal injury may cause internal bleeding or leakage of gut contents, which are often not obvious immediately. On the mountain you can do little to stop whatever mischief is going on inside the abdomen, but keen observation will alert you to the gravity of the injury. Call help early to give the victim the chance of reaching a surgeon with all speed.

How? (Structure)

The abdomen is a cavity housing twenty-eight feet of gut and several vital organs (liver, kidneys, spleen, bladder), each with a rich blood supply. The entire cavity is lined by peritoneum, a thin but very sensitive membrane that also wraps itself round each of the organs. The slippery surface of the peritoneum allows the abdominal organs to slide over each other, expanding and contracting without friction. The peritoneum registers pain when stretched or irritated by spilt blood or acid gut contents.

A. Open Wounds

In the rare event of serious injury to the abdomen, intestines may protrude from the wound — a horrifying sight. Do not try to push them back inside the abdomen, but cover the wound with a clean, preferably sterile, damp dressing until the casualty reaches hospital. If the instrument that caused the injury is still in the wound, leave it there as it may be plugging a hole, and removing it could start a rush of bleeding.

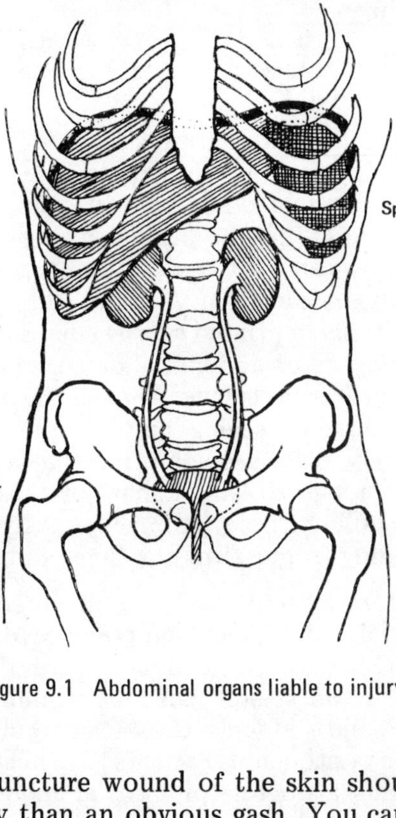

Figure 9.1 Abdominal organs liable to injury

A small puncture wound of the skin should cause far more anxiety than an obvious gash. You can only guess whether the instrument has just nicked the skin and penetrated muscle or whether it has entered the abdominal cavity and pierced a soft internal organ or viscus. Most surgeons will assume that a puncture wound has penetrated the abdominal cavity until proved otherwise and operate forthwith to explore for internal damage. A long sharp object, like a knife, which punctures the skin can be withdrawn leaving barely a mark; a deeply punctured viscus can seal over temporarily but may leak blood or gut contents into the abdominal cavity later with fatal results.

B. Closed Injury

Signs of closed injury may be few; suspicion is your strongest weapon in making a diagnosis.

If the chest is injured always look for an abdominal injury as well. When the lower ribs are fractured the underlying abdominal organ (i.e. liver on the right and spleen on the left) may be pierced by a broken rib end. Even a mild blow can rupture an internal organ so beware of bruising on the abdomen. A bruise showing the fabric pattern of clothing imprinted on the skin is a very significant sign because some abdominal organs must have been tightly squeezed between the skin and the bony spine or pelvis. Many surgeons seeing 'pattern bruising' will operate immediately on the assumption that a compressing force strong enough to leave a mark on the skin is likely to rupture a hollow viscus (stomach, intestines, bladder) or cause bleeding from a firm one (liver, kidney, spleen).

A word of extreme caution — blunt injury to certain organs, especially the spleen and possibly to the kidneys and liver, is liable to cause bleeding beneath the enfolding capsule, which can stretch without warning signs. The pressure rises and suddenly the capsule bursts releasing blood into the peritoneum. Patients have been sent home after consulting a doctor for a trivial abdominal injury only to collapse and die without warning from a massive haemorrhage caused by a delayed rupture of the spleen.

A fractured pelvis may injure the bladder or urethra, and cause much hidden blood loss.

Blood or spilt gut contents lying in the abdominal cavity irritate the peritoneum causing symptoms. If untreated, frank infection (peritonitis) may occur.

On the mountain you can give little active treatment to cure someone with a severe abdominal injury. But your observations, written down on the spot and handed to the receiving surgeon as soon as the casualty reaches hospital, may be lifesaving.

Ask.

The site of the injury gives a clue to the underlying organ that may be damaged. The nature of the object causing the injury and the way the accident happened (e.g. falling across a rock or onto the pick of an ice-axe), may suggest the type of the injury.

Moderate pain may be the casualty's only complaint; if it worsens steadily — beware. Usually pain is felt in the centre of the abdomen but it may spread to other regions. Vomiting is an important sign of abdominal mischief; note the colour and contents of the vomit and keep a sample if possible.

Blood or gut contents coming into contact with the under surface of the diaphragm (the domed muscle sheet separating abdomen and chest) may irritate the peritoneum supplied by the phrenic nerve and pain will be referred to the tip of the shoulder, an area which the phrenic nerve also serves after it divides high up in the neck. If a patient with a suspected abdominal injury lies with his body tipped slightly head down he may complain of pain in one or both shoulders, because the spilled gut contents or blood will trickle towards the diaphragm. This is a useful and simple diagnostic test.

Look.

— Shock is *the* sign of internal bleeding. Head injury patients usually do not become shocked; so if an injured climber is pale, sweaty and cold with a rapid feeble pulse look to the abdomen for the cause of shock.

— Vomiting often results from peritonitis. Fresh blood in the vomit is most likely due to blood from an associated nose or mouth injury trickling into the stomach.

— Peritonitis causes the abdomen to be held quite still during breathing and only the lower chest moves; normal quiet breathing is done with the diaphragm and its movement can be seen in the upper abdomen.

— Blood in the urine suggests damage to kidneys or bladder; blood at the end of the penis suggests urethral injury.

Feel.

Gently press on the casualty's abdomen with the flat of your hand, but not hard enough to cause pain. The abdominal muscles will become tense 'guarding' the injured organs and resisting the pressure of your hand. Later on the muscles may feel rigid, like pressing on a board. Further pressure causes pain, so desist but note the sign nonetheless.

Act.

— Reassure the casualty. If he is flippant about an injury that you suspect is not trivial, warn him of the dangers of not heeding your advice. He may not be aware of the possibility of a temporarily sealed wound or a delayed rupture of the spleen.

— Rest him completely. If you are likely to reach hospital within a couple of hours don't let him drink but just moisten his lips with water. If far from help, allow only sips by mouth because he may vomit. He may need an emergency anaesthetic as soon as he reaches hospital; but fluid in the stomach is the anaesthetist's problem, not yours, and he has means at his disposal for dealing with it. A dry patient is often a restless one.

— Write all your observations on paper. Make a half-hourly record of his pulse.

— Keep a small sample of all excretions (vomit, faeces,

urine), which can be tested in hospital later. Observation with the naked eye may not yield as much information as the microscope.

— Take a sample of blood (10 ml.) if you have a syringe and needle. It need not be put in a sterile bottle, and if it clots it does not matter as the decanted serum is all that is wanted for cross-matching blood ready for transfusion. If you wait until the casualty is shocked before taking blood, it may be very hard to get from collapsed veins.

— Treat.

Shock. (q.v.)

Pain. Morphine will relieve pain and allay anxiety, but it tends to make the person vomit. Do not give morphine if you are likely to reach a doctor within two hours as it may mask pain that will point to the diagnosis, but do not withold it if he faces a long carry.

Infection. Blood is an ideal growth medium for bugs, and spilt intestinal juices are teeming with bacteria, so the stage is set for infection. If you have a long time to wait before reaching help, give a large dose of broad spectrum antibiotic by intramuscular injection.

Fractured Pelvis

Falling from a height is the commonest cause of a climber crushing the ring of the pelvic bones. Because the pelvis is surrounded by many muscles and hollow spaces a severe fracture may not be obvious, and the patient's only complaint may be of pain round the hips and difficulty in walking. Several pints of blood can seep away into the tissues unnoticed before the casualty suddenly collapses from shock. He may rupture his urethra or bladder (see over).

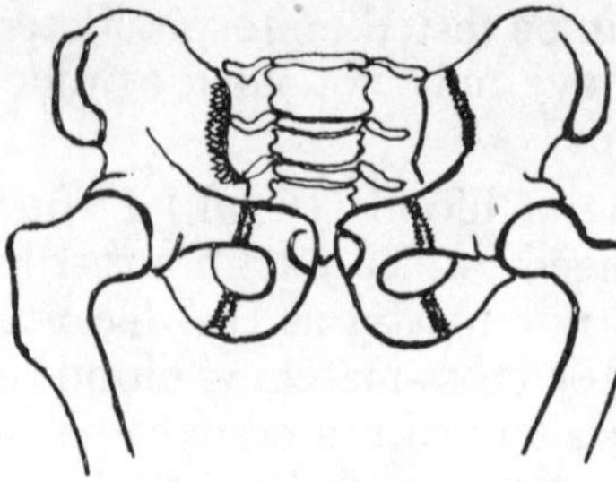

Figure 9.2 Pelvis fracture sites

Act.

Pad the crutch with soft wool clothing and put a firm supporting binder round the upper thighs; bandage the knees and feet together to prevent the legs moving on the pelvis. Treat the casualty for pain and carry him gently off the mountain on a stretcher.

Rupture of the Urethra or Bladder

After bleeding, the most serious problem arising from a fractured pelvis is rupture of the urethra or, less commonly, the bladder. The urethra is torn when the fractured segment of pelvis, to which it is tethered, is pulled apart. The urethra can also be injured by falling astride a rock. These injuries are almost exclusively confined to men.

Look.

Blood appears at the end of the penis and the crutch is bruised by the blow or because of seeping blood. The bladder may become distended some hours later and be very uncomfortable. The swollen bladder is often impossible to see but it can be felt above the pubic bone.

The patient will not be able to pass urine so traditional exhortations not to do so are pointless. Urine spreads up into the muscle planes of the lower abdomen instead of passing down the damaged urethra. The blood and urine that pools may become dangerously infected.

Act.

Give a broad spectrum antibiotic immediately. Nothing else need be done for 24 hours; absolutely no harm can come from inactivity and a lot of meddlesome damage may be avoided. If you are far from help and the patient's bladder becomes swollen after waiting for 24 hours, plunge a sterile needle through the cleansed skin of the abdominal wall one inch (2 cm.) above the pubic bone in the mid-line, and let the urine spurt out. If the needle can be fixed in position with tape, it is best to do so and to let the urine drain away into dressings or attach a plastic tube to it as a drain. Otherwise the bladder will have to be needled as often as it swells up. Do not try to pass a catheter into the urethra. Leave any further intervention to a waterworks specialist.

10

Major and Minor Burns

Rope friction burns of the hands, neck and back can occur when trying to hold a falling climber; camping and fires go hand in hand; burns and scalds by cooking pans, boiling fat and hot liquids are common. But the greatest hazard is a gas stove explosion in the confined space of a tent or camping van, causing skin burns from lighted fabric and burns of the lungs from inhaling hot gases. Liquid gas is heavier than air; when it escapes unburnt from a cylinder it settles on the floor and may lie unnoticed because it has no appreciable smell. Another hazard of cooking within a confined space without adequate ventilation is carbon monoxide poisoning (see p. 126).

Minor burns are a painful nuisance. A major burn is a serious threat to life with consequences that stretch far beyond the local burn wound. The degree of burning is assessed by the area of body surface that is burnt, irrespective of depth.

Major burns in adults involve more than 15% of the body surface area.

Major burns in children involve more than 10% of the body surface area (because a child has greater body surface in relation to weight).

Percentage body surface area is measured by the 'Rule of 9's' (Wallace),

or by the palm of the patient's hand (not your own) which = 1% of the body surface area.

Major burns cause two main problems, tissue destruc-

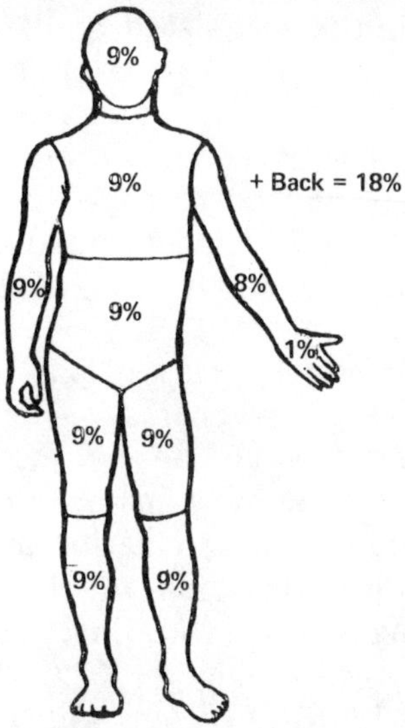

Figure 10.1 Rule of 9s

tion and loss of fluid. These combine together to cause shock, similar to the shock that follows severe bleeding, which must not be confused with the emotion, fear, pain and fainting that may result from the burning accident (though these may compound and worsen clinical shock).

How?

i. Fluid loss. Damaged capillaries dilate and leak plasma in proportion to the area of the burn. Plasma is the fluid portion of the blood in which red and white corpuscles are suspended; serum is plasma from which the protein, fibrinogen, has been separated in the process of clotting. Plasma exudes from the raw surface, forms large blisters under the outer epithelial layers of the skin and collects round the burn in tissues which swell severely. Some red cells are trapped in the coagulated skin and destroyed by the heat; others pass on into the circulation and fragment later because scorching renders them more fragile. The end products of broken-down blood cells lodge in the kidney, which may be damaged by them, or they may escape in the urine giving it a reddish-brown colour — a serious sign. The destruction of red cells causes anaemia.

The body compensates for loss of plasma from a minor burn by natural defence mechanisms. Fluid is withdrawn from regions where it is not needed instantly, vessels in the periphery of the skin and in the gut clamp down so blood pools in the central circulation and thirst is compulsive, making up for some of the lost fluid. But too free drinking causes vomiting, so it pays to be moderate.

After a major burn the victim will become clinically shocked when his body is no longer able to cope with the loss of plasma, so fluid must be given by intravenous infusion ('drip') to raise the plasma volume to normal levels. A person who has bled severely soon becomes shocked in proportion to the blood lost; but 'burns shock' develops slowly over several hours so the casualty may appear deceptively well immediately after the accident and then 'go off' over the next 24–36 hours. The burnt area must be measured accurately and the volume of fluid to be replaced must be assessed according to a formula, tempered by judging the patient's condition. Guesswork has no place in the management of severe burns.

ii. Tissue destruction. A burn is a wound. Skin cells are destroyed and dead tissue releases poisonous substances that worsen the state of shock. The depth of tissue destroyed is important, not so much in the early stages when the victim is most in danger of dying of shock, but in determining the time that the wound will take to heal, and whether skin grafting will be necessary.

For practical purposes a burn is either superficial or deep.

a. Superficial (partial thickness). The burn involves only the skin of the epidermis and part of the dermis where the hair follicles and sweat and sebaceous glands lie. Unharmed epithelial cells in the bottom of the wound rapidly spread to form new skin. No potions or poultices speed healing, but infection delays it and may convert a superficial burn into a deep one. Superficial burns usually heal by themselves in 7–21 days.

b. Deep (full thickness). All the epithelial cells are destroyed. Nerves also die so pain is no longer felt. Exuded plasma and coagulated tissue form a slough which, if left open to the air, hardens into a dry crust. Healing

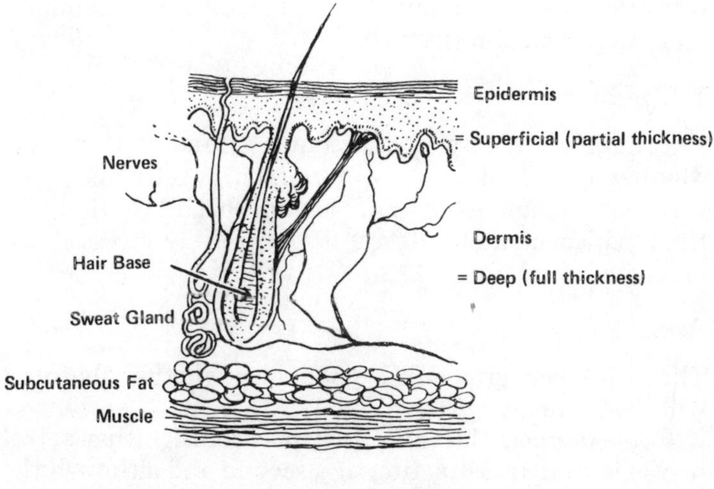

Figure 10.2 Skin layers

goes on under the crust which eventually separates leaving a raw area of scar tissue. This may subsequently contract owing to fibrosis. Early skin grafting can prevent the hideous and disabling deformities that are a common sequel to major burns.

A major burn presents four main problems:

1. The burn wound.
2. The airway.
3. Pain.
4. Fluid loss.

You will have great difficulty in managing a major burn out in the wilds. The ideal treatment is explained here, although it may appear far beyond your scope. If you have a clear understanding of the burn problems you may be able to apply at least some basic principles to save the life of the victim and to keep his injury to a minimum. Just because you are in a remote mountain range several days or weeks away from help, do not despair nor give up trying. Your ingenuity and common sense may well win through.

1. The Burn Wound

The immediate care of the burn wound is the same whether it is a major or a minor burn; refinements in treatment come later. You cannot begin to think of fluid replacement until you have carefully assessed the extent of the burn.

Ask.

The story will give you a good idea whether the burn will heal quickly or not.

For example, the flash of flame from igniting petrol or gas is over in a fraction of a second and although the skin is burned brown or black, the burn will be superficial and heal in 7-10 days. Explosions in a confined space such as a tent are extremely serious because hot gases are inhaled, burning the air passages and lungs. If clothing catches fire the flame will continue to burn the skin for several seconds causing a deep burn which will take weeks or months to heal. Many synthetic fibres burn rapidly and inflict severe injury. Wool delays flame from reaching the skin but it encourages boiling water to stick so increasing the scalding time, and thus burning deeply. However boiling water and hot fat poured onto bare skin will usually cause only superficial damage. But the flames from a frying pan that has caught fire will burn deeply if they play on bare skin for more than a second or two. Chemical burns from acid or lime, if recognized quickly and washed copiously, are rarely deep. Electrical burns are always deep and very slow to heal, especially where the current enters and leaves the body; however, an electric flash causes a superficial burn.

Look.

a. At the patient. Is he breathing with difficulty?

Is he in pain?

Is he shocked?

If any of these applies start the appropriate treatment.

b. At the burn.

— In order to examine the full extent of the burn, remove any charred clothing. If it sticks to the skin leave in place, or bleeding may start, and anyway burned cloth will be sterile from the heat.

— Assess the burnt skin area by the 'rule of 9's' and decide whether the burn is major (more than 15% adult, 10% child) or minor.

— Estimate the depth of the burn and draw a diagram to show the areas of deep and superficial burning, that will help to show the progress of subsequent healing.

The colour of the skin is a poor guide to the depth of a burn; it only tells you the temperature of the burning agents which you will already know from the story.

Feel.

— The 'Pinprick Test' is the best way to determine the depth of a burn. If the patient can feel a prick with a sterile pin firm enough to draw blood (light touch is not enough) the nerves in the deep layers of the skin are undamaged. Absent feeling of pain is a sign of deep burning.

— The 'Pressure Test' is useful in scalds where the skin looks pink. If the skin feels leathery and firm on pressure, it is deeply burned. If the colour returns quickly when you remove your pressing finger the burn is less than deep.

Act.

a. Cool. Plunge the part immediately into cold water for at least 10 minutes. Cooling relieves pain, reduces swelling and may diminish the depth of the burn. Do not smear it with butter or 'burn creams' which confuse the picture and make dressings stick fast, or antibiotic creams which encourage the growth of resistant bacteria.

b. Clean. Remove burnt clothes and dead tissue and wash with soap and water or an antiseptic solution such as cetrimide and chlorhexidine. Chemical burns (especially lime in the eyes) must be irrigated with plain water for at least ten minutes.

c. Cover. A dressing acts as a mechanical barrier to infection and absorbs the exudate from the wound allowing it to dry and start healing. Cover the wound with a clean, preferably sterile, dry linen or non-stick dressing, or two layers of greasy tulle gras gauze. Over the first dressing place a layer of cotton gauze which lets fluid pass through its meshwork. Then apply a pad of absorbent cotton wool to soak up the exuded fluid. The dressing must extend at least a handsbreadth beyond the edge of the burnt area. Finally, wrap a crepe bandage evenly over the dressing, firm enough to keep it in place but not so tight as to restrict blood flow. If you have no immediate chance of reaching help this burn dressing can be left in place for up to a week provided it remains dry. But as soon as plasma soaks through the dressing, repack it with plenty of absorbent wool. Undo the dressing completely and start again if it smells unpleasant, if there is pussy discharge, if pain and redness develop in skin away from the burn, or if the patient's temperature rises for no explicable reason. These are the signs of infection.

d. Blisters. Puncture blisters with a sterile needle or blade as they will break anyway. Remove any dead skin; carefully lancing on the first day can be quite painless. Pay scrupulous attention to cleanliness, as infection can easily creep into the open wound you have made. If you wait till blisters have broken by themselves and are infected, 'deroofing' is exquisitely painful.

e. Drugs.

— Antibiotics. If you suspect infection give a broad spectrum antibiotic, preferably one of the penicillin family, for at least 10 days.

— Analgesics. The burn itself may give little pain, but changing dressings can be agonizing, so give a strong painkiller before you start.

— Tetanus toxoid. Always give a booster dose of tetanus toxoid to a major burn.

f. Exposure to air. In hospital the best treatment for a major burn may be to leave it open to the air so that it dries, forming a hard crusting scab that keeps out bacteria, and under which healing proceeds. However, out on the hill it is unlikely this method will be suitable. While trying to evacuate the victim dressings will be more convenient.

All your treatment of the burn wound is aimed towards keeping it clean and avoiding infection so that it can heal as quickly as possible. In hospital skin grafting may be needed to treat areas of deep burning and if the wound is clean this can be done soon after arrival.

Special Burn Sites

a. Face. Most face burns can be left exposed to the air. But the lax tissues of the face swell and may close the patient's eyes, so reassure him that he is not going blind. Make sure his eyes are not damaged; while they are closed an antibiotic cream put in twice a day will prevent infection.

b. Eyelids. Burnt lids may retract exposing the cornea (window of the eye) which quickly becomes ulcerated if not kept moist with cream, which remains in the eye longer than drops.

c. Eyes. Corneal burns are uncommon because you usually blink before the flame reaches the eye. But if corrosive chemicals (e.g. lime) get into the eye wash thoroughly with water until you are sure every particle has gone, and put homatropine 1% drops and an antibiotic cream into the eye twice daily and keep it covered with a pad and bandage.

d. Hands. Burnt hands form nasty contracture deformities *after* healing unless they are kept moving *while* healing. Cover the whole hand liberally with antibiotic cream and put it into a plastic bag. Encourage the patient to exercise his fingers continually to prevent the skin hardening and the fingers becoming stiff. By elevating the hand swelling is reduced. The patient with a 'bagged' hand can do a lot for himself without pain; a mitten over the top prevents the bag tearing and looks less distasteful.

e. Circumferential burns. Deep burns of the circumference of the neck, chest, limbs or fingers harden and the scab may contract like a ring and cut off the blood supply or restrict movement.

Check by pin-prick that pain sensation is absent in the burnt hand. Then take a knife and cut deeply through the charred skin till the wound spreads apart. This apparently drastic treatment is simple yet vital to prevent obstruction of breathing or serious damage to limbs. It is completely free of pain in the burned area but to be effective you must cut beyond the very top and bottom of the band down into the painful unburned zone, which may bleed. This is most important with a deep burn round the wrist where the hand is unburned. If the cuts are adequate, you will see the swollen veins and mottled blue colour of the skin return to a healthy pink. Where fingers are burned deeply to the tips all round, it is doubtful if splitting the burn makes much difference.

2. The Airway

Pay meticulous attention to the airway. To lose a victim of burning from airway block is tragic because it is usually avoidable.

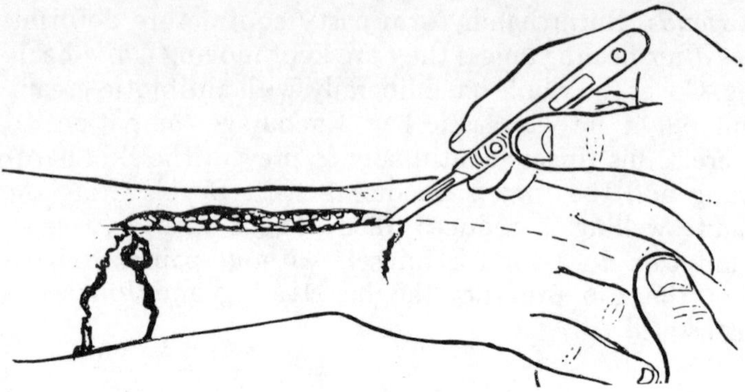

Figure 10.3 Cutting into a burnt hand

Look.

a. Face. Blue, cyanosed lips suggest airway block or breathing difficulty. If the lips, tongue, or the hairs of the nostrils are scorched after an explosion you can presume the casualty has inhaled burning gas. The larynx and trachea are bound to swell and this may lead to airway block. If the lungs are burned pneumonia will almost certainly develop.

b. Chest. A firm hard crust, like a breastplate of armour, may form over his chest and splint his breathing.

Listen.

A husky voice suggests that the larynx is swollen; croaking stridor heralds a serious block. Bubbly noises in the chest indicate a collection of fluid (pulmonary oedema) or the onset of pneumonia.

Act.

If in doubt about the airway pass an endotracheal tube early rather than late. When the casualty reaches hospital a tracheotomy may be needed but beware of doing this in the field as it can be a very difficult operation.

When a tight crust limits breathing make long cuts through the full thickness of the burnt skin to relieve his breathing (see opposite).

3. Pain

Not only is pain very unpleasant to suffer, but it aggravates shock; so reassure the victim and treat him with adequate doses of analgesic drugs. Morphine will probably be needed in the first instance, but there are other choices of drugs for long term pain relief should you be worried about addiction.

Give small doses of the chosen drug directly into a vein, repeated as frequently as necessary. With one large injection into a muscle the drug may lie stagnant because the state of shock temporarily reduces blood flow; when it does eventually pick up, a slug of the drug will be released suddenly, and powerfully depress the breathing.

Pain is registered by nerve endings in the epidermis, so the superficial skin layers must be intact if pain is felt, yet serious burns may be surprisingly free from pain.

4. Fluid Loss

Plasma is the main fluid lost after a burn; it must be replaced to avoid shock.

Look.

Determine the surface area of the burn by the 'Rule of 9's', paying attention only to the area of burning. The crucial question is "to drip or not to drip". Major burns need transfusion, minor burns do not. Although we take a figure of 15% as the major burn area at which to start transfusion for an adult, healthy people will survive without transfusion from burns twice and possibly three times this area. So do not despair if you are unable to give intravenous fluids.

Act.

After a minor burn the patient can make up his lost fluid by his own body resources and by drinking. Give small amounts of fluid by mouth, otherwise he may vomit, and give frequent sips rather than big gulps. The best drink is a solution made by adding one teaspoon of salt and one teaspoon of bicarbonate of soda to one litre of water.

After a major burn a 'drip' is the best way of restoring fluid. If you are really out on a limb with no chance of giving fluid into a vein, a safe method is to give it by way of the rectum. Insert a greased rubber tube with a funnel attached about four inches past the anus and run fluid in at such a rate that the patient can retain it. The circulation cannot be overloaded in this way.

If you have facilities for transfusion and are in a camp where the regime can be carried out, choose a big vein as the 'drip' may have to be continued for several days (see transfusion p. 48). While you are setting up the drip take blood into a plain tube, for cross-matching later. The best replacement fluid is dried human plasma reconstituted with sterile water, as it has all the essential proteins in it; normal saline (salt solution) will do temporarily.

Plasma should be given at a rate calculated by the following formula:

$$\% \text{ burn} \times \tfrac{1}{2} \text{ patient's weight in kg.} = \text{millilitres per 'period'}$$

The periods of time in hours after the burn are: 4, 4, 4, 6, 6, 12. For example an eleven stone man (70 kg.) with all of both arms, face, chest and part of his back burned, has about 40% of his skin surface involved, and will need: $40 \times 70/2 = 1{,}400$ mls. ($2\frac{1}{2}$ pints) of plasma in each period of time.

At least twice as much saline will be needed as plasma because saline flows fast through damaged tissue and does not maintain the blood circulation as well as plasma. Fortunately the kidney corrects quite big errors for us.

A casualty who is short of fluid will show the following signs:—

— Restless behaviour; especially true of children.

— Pale cold skin. A cold nose is a bad sign. The patient should be pink and warm; his big toe, when squeezed, should blanch for a second or so and then the colour should return quickly on releasing the pressure (the big toe test).

— Rapid pulse. It feels weak and thready against your fingers. The force of his pulse will rise as he overcomes his shock, and its rate will slow down.

— Low urine output. Collect all the urine he passes and measure it over a 12 hour period, noticing whether it is dark and concentrated, or pale and dilute. He should pass more than 25 ml. (one fluid ounce) of urine each hour, indicating that the kidneys are getting an adequate blood flow.

— Sluggish gut movement. If shock paralyses the intestines the patient may vomit. He feels thirsty because his gut is not absorbing water adequately, and his belly may become acutely distended.

— Dry furred tongue. This usually becomes moist after two or three days when he will be able to eat and drink again.

Carry.

Finally, do not delay evacuating the victim to hospital as he will travel best immediately after the accident and before shock sets in.

Keep your cool and do the best you can according to these guidelines in the time while you are waiting, before he becomes shocked. Reassure him that you are doing all you can to reach help urgently. Do not brush off his questions, such as 'Is it serious?' or 'Will I be in hospital for long?': give a full reply to the best of your ability. Let us hope optimism is warranted, but if you have done your best, that is the maximum you can hope for.

11

Bone and Joint Trauma

Injuries to bones and joints are usually due to the hazards of tripping and falling on rough or icy ground.

A. FRACTURES

To fracture means to break, no more no less; but a 'fractured femur' sounds much more serious and mysterious than a 'broken thigh'. Just as a chair leg will break if you knock, bend, twist, pull or crush it beyond a certain limit, so will bones break or crack; the difference is that wood is inert but bone is living. Bones mend and wounds heal by following similar patterns. Fractures are described according to the shape of the broken bone ends; for practical purposes of mountain care the important distinction is between 'open' and 'closed' fractures. But remember that the entire limb needs treatment whether of a hairline bone crack, the soft tissues surrounding the injured bone or a major break.

The skin of an *open* fracture has been breached; in *closed* fractures the skin is intact. Whether the skin is broken from within by the jagged ends or by the breaking force from outside, the underlying fractured bone is open to infection, which delays healing and may progress to osteomyelitis — a dreaded complication.

All fractures need splinting to prevent the broken fragments moving against each other, causing pain and further damage to neighbouring muscles, nerves and blood vessels. Stable fractures, where there is no movement, may become unstable if inadequately supported.

How?

Bone is a plastic living tissue that makes a rigid framework to support muscles and ligaments attached to it and to protect the contents of the skull and thorax. The dried skeleton in an anatomy school is not typical bone, which normally has a rich blood supply, as can be seen on the butcher's slab. In the central core of a long bone lies the marrow, a loose matrix of spicules with pools of soft blood-forming cells. The cortex forms the weight-bearing rigid outer casing surrounded by a tough membrane of periosteum to which muscles, tendons and ligaments are attached. Periosteum is rich in nerve fibres and registers most of the pain of a broken bone.

a. General.

Shock. The casualty may be 'shocked' because of severe pain or worry about the outcome of his accident — a forced bivouac or rescue call-out. But he may also be in a state of physiological shock from loss of blood into the tissues causing a low blood pressure and rapid pulse. A severely fractured thigh or lower leg may contain 2 litres of blood (i.e. 1/5 of the total blood volume). Bleeding comes from the marrow cavity, vessels in the periosteum and surrounding muscle and tissues torn by the jagged bone ends. With multiple fractures and open wounds the blood loss may be considerably more.

b. Local

i. Bony damage.

Ask.

— Where does it hurt? Most fractures cause a dull ache rather than severe pain. When bone fragments move suddenly causing the ends to grate or the periosteum to tear, they become very painful.

— Can he move the injured part? He may 'guard' it because of pain. Never forcibly move a limb you suspect may be broken. Grating bone ends may confirm your diagnosis; this brutality is inexcusable as it not only causes pain and worsens the shock, but it may shift an acceptable position of the fragments. If the bone is broken right across, the limb beyond may be abnormally mobile, like a flail, and such movement will be exceedingly painful.

Look.

Remove clothing to let you have a good look at the injured limb and its normal opposite, if necessary cutting the clothes away. Whenever you suspect damage in a paired bone, compare the two sides and a slight swelling or deformity will become obvious at a glance.

a. Swelling. Bleeding from the bone end and from torn vessels in the surrounding soft tissues causes swelling. Several pints of blood may be released into the tissues when a large bone (e.g. the thigh) is broken. Bruising appears later when the discoloration from shed blood seeps through to the skin.

b. Deformity. If the bone is angled where no joint exists you can be sure of a fracture. Severe deformity suggests serious damage.

Feel.

Tenderness. Gentle pressure over a break, even a very small one, causes pain. Tenderness is an invariable sign of a fracture; it makes the casualty grimace so always look at his face when you are examining his foot (and any other bones).

ii. Associated damage.
Damage to the soft parts around the bone may be more important than the bone injury itself.

a. Blood vessels. Not only may vessels be torn and bleed, but pinching a main artery in the fracture will embarrass the circulation to the whole limb. Swelling of the tissues and the resulting tenseness can hamper blood flow so the pulse may be difficult or impossible to feel. Usually the blood flow is adequate if the skin beyond the injury is warm and pink, but beware if it goes blue or white and remains blanched after pressing on it.

b. Skin. Swelling makes the skin weak through stretching. If the skin is breached a closed fracture becomes an open one. Any bruising or damage to the skin renders it less elastic and therefore weaker.

c. Nerves. Numbness, loss of pain and feeling, and paralysis are signs that nerves have been damaged and should be noted. Nerve pressure is not urgent and will be dealt with later by a surgeon at leisure.

Act.

If you suspect an injured climber has broken a bone, release any tight clothing and avoid putting on tight bandages, both of which restrict the circulation.

Splinting is the key to handling broken bones, since once an unstable bone is held firmly it can be handled painlessly; the fracture now being stable, further damage is avoided. Complete immobilization is only possible in a plaster cast; the best you can hope for on the mountain is to hold it reasonably still.

Splinting

a. Open wounds. Open fractures, where the skin is broken, need special care before splinting. Remove clothing from the wound and clear away dirt and debris. Wash the wound with soap and water or an antiseptic solution, then cover it with a sterile dressing held in place with loose tape. Use a large pack firmly bandaged into place to stop bleeding, but beware of bandaging too tightly as you may damage the skin by pressure.

Give anti-tetanus protection (see p. 176) and an antibiotic as soon as possible to stave off infection, especially osteomyelitis.

b. Deformity. If deformity is corrected first it is easier to apply a splint properly. This is safe and harmless provided it can be done without undue pain to or resistance from the casualty. Straightening a limb may cause an absent pulse to reappear because pressure on the blood vessel is released.

So correct the deformity before splinting:—

a. if the bone is severely angled and in danger of stretching or pinching blood vessels or nerves.

b. if the skin is taut and blanched, suggesting that its blood supply is threatened by a projecting fragment of bone under it.

Handle broken bones gently. Sudden movement causes pain so the casualty will tighten his muscles to prevent further movement, and this muscle spasm itself is painful. Local anaesthetic injected directly into the fracture site will ease the pain before handling the bone, but it may remove 'protective pain' and a sharp fragment can puncture the skin from within, creating an open fracture.

Encourage the casualty to relax by quietly explaining what you are going to do so he will not be taken by surprise. A shot of morphia or a large nip of alcohol given before manipulating the bone will both ease the pain and give a sense of relaxed well-being. Two people can hold a limb better than one. Handle it 'all in one piece', both moving together so the fracture is not disturbed.

It is sometimes helpful to pull on the broken limb in order to straighten it before attempting to move the broken fragment to its correct position. Take a firm grasp well away from the broken bone on uninjured skin while your assistant holds the limb near the trunk. Gently, firmly and steadily increase your pull, taking plenty of time over it. Watch the casualty's face all the time, not your hands, as you will not learn anything from them. If the manoeuvre seems to be unduly painful, keep on pulling for a longer time before trying to move the bone ends. Discretion will have to make you decide when the time has come to stop hurting him.

Once you have separated the grating bone ends you will be able to restore them to their natural position ready for splinting. If you can make a broken bone comfortable and avoid further damage without splinting,

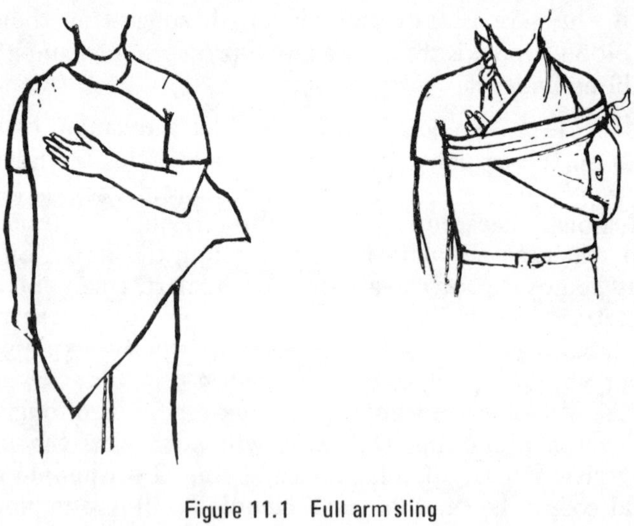

Figure 11.1 Full arm sling

do so. But if you must splint because the fracture is unstable, the rule is — reduce movement in the joints above and below the break. Common advice is to splint the limb 'where it lies', before moving the casualty so that he can then be moved onto a stretcher without pain. But if you are in an awkward and difficult place on the mountainside he may become impossibly immobile by being trussed up; unsplinted he may be able to help you move himself to a safer position.

Before splinting, pad below any weight-bearing points (e.g. heels) and between bony prominences (e.g. ankles) with loose cloth or wool or a ring pad. Fill the hollows under the knees. Tie bindings so they hold the part still but not tight enough to embarrass the blood supply. Always leave toes and finger tips open to view, but lightly covered for protection, so you can watch their colour and warmth. Take swift appropriate action if they become pale, blue or cold.

Many things can be used for splints.

a. The most available splint is the body itself. A broken arm can be strapped to the chest and a broken leg can be bandaged to the opposite uninjured leg.

b. Improvised. Bark peeled from birch, poplar, alder or any hardwood and lined with moss or grass makes an excellent splint. Newspaper can be rolled into a rigid tube, cardboard can be bent to form a gutter and angled where necessary. A tree branch or an ice-axe may be used for a leg splint. A stout sapling trimmed correctly makes a satisfactory arm crutch.

c. Malleable. Certain splinting materials can be bent to conform to the shape of the limb. Kramer wire is made of criss-crossed wire, and there are plastic compounds that soften with heat and harden on cooling.

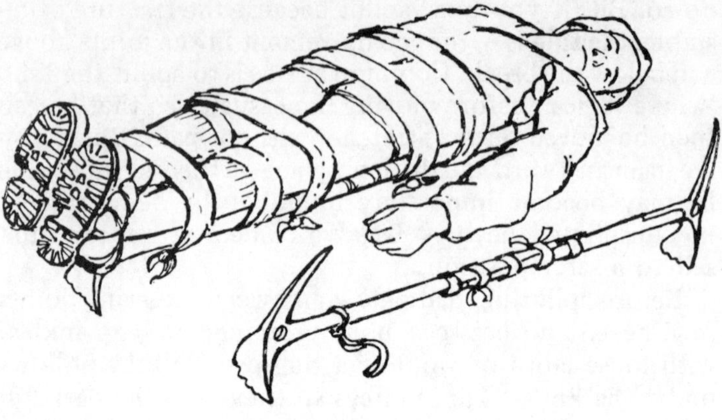

Figure 11.2 Ice-axe leg splint

d. Inflatable. The limb is put into a double-skinned tube that is blown up to conform to the shape of the limb. Some inflatable splints wrap around the limb and are then closed by a zip-fastener or 'Velcro' self-adhesive

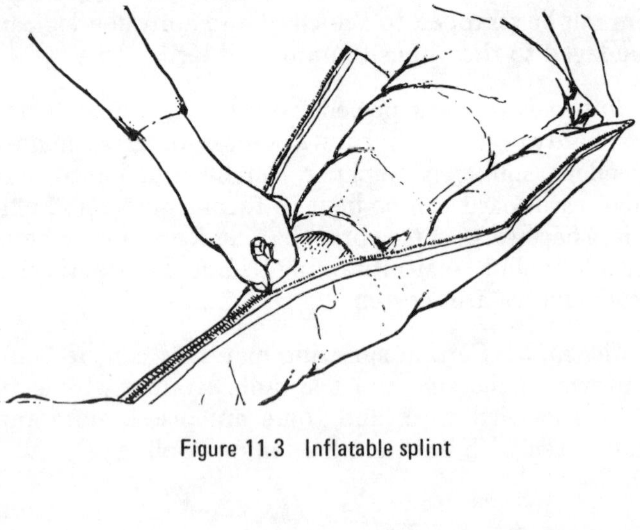

Figure 11.3 Inflatable splint

material. These splints are frequently criticised on the grounds that they may be blown up too tight and cut off the blood supply. No harm will come if they are inflated by mouth so they can still be easily indented with finger pressure. Always leave the fingers and toes open for inspection. Inflatable splints are convenient as they fold small and can be put on over clothing but different sizes are needed for arms and legs. With careful handling they should not puncture though this becomes more likely with age.

e. Traction. The Thomas leg splint has not been bettered over the century since it was invented.

While an assistant pulls steadily on the casualty's foot, thread the ring over the limb until it comes up against the bone on the highest part of the inner thigh. The leg rests on supporting slings secured with safety pins be-between the arms of the splint. Tie an 'ankle-hitch' over the boot with a triangular bandage and secure it to the cross end-piece of the splint. You can increase the pull

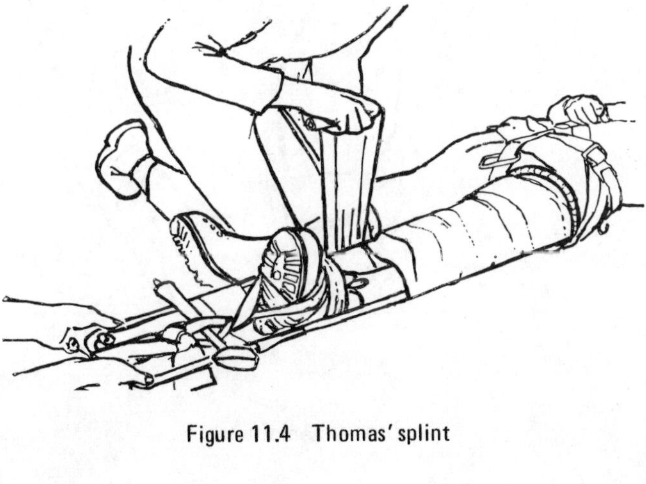

Figure 11.4 Thomas' splint

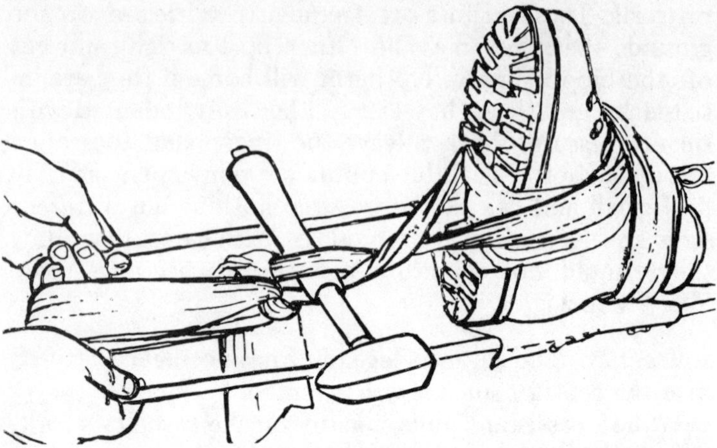

Figure 11.5 Ankle-hitch windlass traction

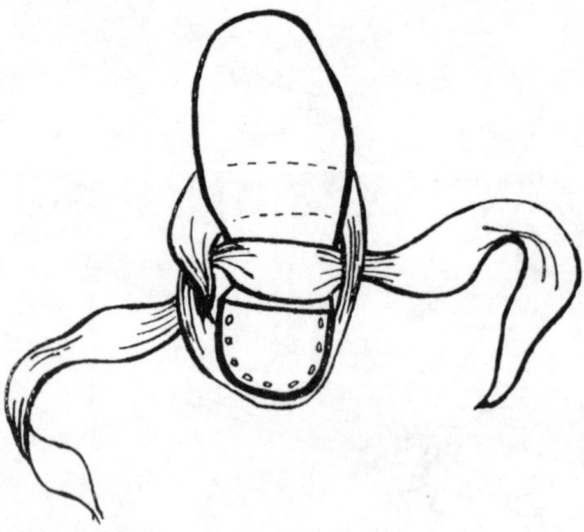

Figure 11.6 Ankle-hitch

on the leg by windlassing this bandage, but beware not to overtighten it. After a while the casualty may complain of increasing pain around the ankle-hitch, so be prepared to slacken the tension. Remember that when his boot is on you cannot see the colour of his toes nor feel if they are warm or cold.

f. Plaster of Paris (P.o.P.). Plaster sets hard after being wetted, and makes a rigid cast. Emergency packs are made up in a plastic bag with the plaster bandages on rollers. Fill the bag with water (this avoids fuss with bowls) and the plaster is ready to use immediately it has been soaked and most of the water squeezed out. The safest plaster splint is the 'back-slab'. Half a dozen layers are moulded onto the natural contour of the back of the limb, encasing not more than $\frac{3}{4}$ of its circumference so that the remaining gap allows the limb to expand if it swells. The limb should be on slight traction in the normal position of rest. Do not aim at perfection as this plaster is only a temporary splint and a definitive plaster will be put on at hospital.

Never apply plaster directly to the skin; put it on over padding either of wool or the casualty's clothing left in place. Fold any loose ends back so there is no chance of rubbing the skin when the plaster hardens, which happens within a few minutes of being put on. Place a loose bandage of cotton or crepe to hold the plaster slab in place.

Specific Broken Bones

A. Upper limb. In most cases a sling is sufficient to hold the broken arm still until the casualty reaches hospital. A makeshift sling can be made by pinning his sleeve to the shoulder of his jacket, or using an ordinary triangular bandage or a collar and cuff and his bad arm can be held

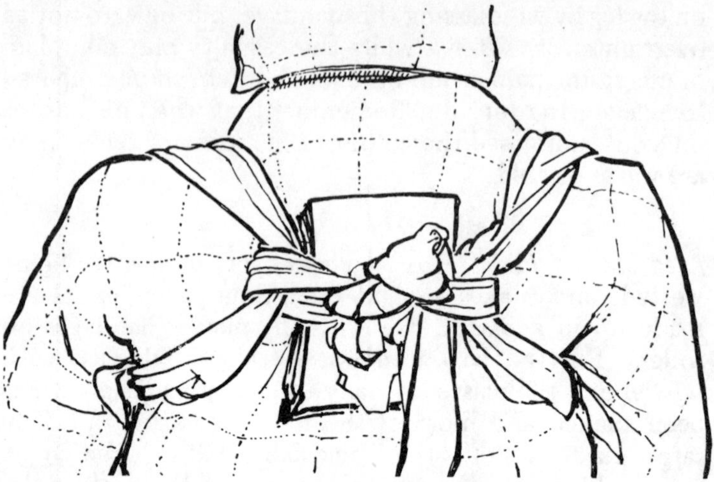

Figure 11.7 Figure-of-8 bandage

and supported by the good one. A swathe made of another triangular bandage or a roll of Elastoplast is bound round the chest over the clothing to hold the arm still.

— Clavicle (collar bone). Usually a sling is adequate, but if the pain is severe a figure-of-8 bandage, with a wad of padding under the cross-over, will brace the shoulders back and prevent the broken ends grating. If the hands go numb or tingle, slacken the bandage.

— Fractures round the elbow. In children these are serious because of the blood vessels and nerves lie close to the bones and may be damaged in an attempt to correct the position, so splint the limb as you find it. If the pulse seems to be absent it is reasonable to try to straighten the elbow in order to restore blood flow.

— Hand. Make a 'boxing glove' by putting a sock or fluffed up handkerchief in the palm of the hand and a bulky crepe bandage round it, leaving out the fingertips for inspection.

— Fingers. Strap the broken finger to its normal neighbour for simple support.

B. Lower limb. After breaking a leg the casualty will be unable to walk and splinting will probably be needed.

— Femur (thigh). Improvise a single splint from armpit to foot made of a long board or wood stake that will stabilize the whole leg. Use masses of padding and secure it with several ties round the chest and above and below the knee. The two legs may be tied together using the sound one as the splint, but it is very uncomfortable for the patient to be tied up so. A Thomas splint is made for the job. It can be used very successfully for any injury from the hip down to the ankle and is valuable even in soft tissue injuries not involving bone where there is massive swelling from hidden bleeding.

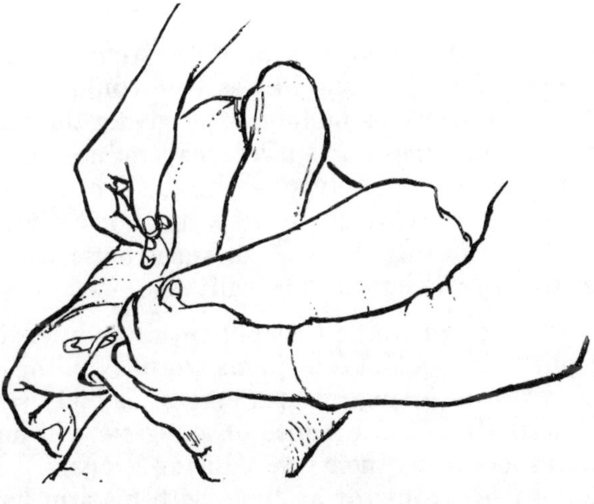

Figure 11.8 Ankle pillow splint

— Tibia (shin-bone). Splint according to the rule that the joint above and below the fracture must be immobilized i.e. from above the knee to the toes.

— Patella (knee-cap). Fix the knee straight with a firm back-slab or splint.

— Ankle. Use heavy wool padding and a firm bandage, or a pillow wrapped round the ankle and secured with safety pins.

B. DISLOCATIONS

Dislocation occurs when the bone end that forms a joint is displaced, tearing the ligaments that hold it in place. The signs are similar to those of a fracture (pain, deformity, swelling, loss of use) but the abnormal position of the joint usually makes the diagnosis obvious. Because nerves and blood vessels are close at hand leave the deformity as it is, provided help can be reached in reasonable time. Splint a dislocated joint above and below the displaced joint.

Out in the wilds you may have to attempt to reduce the dislocation in the same way as you would a fracture. Gentle and continuous pulling, after giving the casualty a pain and apprehension reliever, may reduce the dislocation if done immediately after the accident and before the overlying muscles go into spasm. Once they have tightened up nothing short of an anaesthetic will allow the position of the bones to be shifted.

— Shoulder. If you are on the spot within minutes of the injury put your socked foot in his armpit, pulling on his hand and slowly easing his arm across his body (Hippocrates method). A strong dose of analgesic will help. If this is unsuccessful, then try reducing it again. Lie the casualty on his front for an hour with his arm hanging down to exert a gentle pull by gravity.

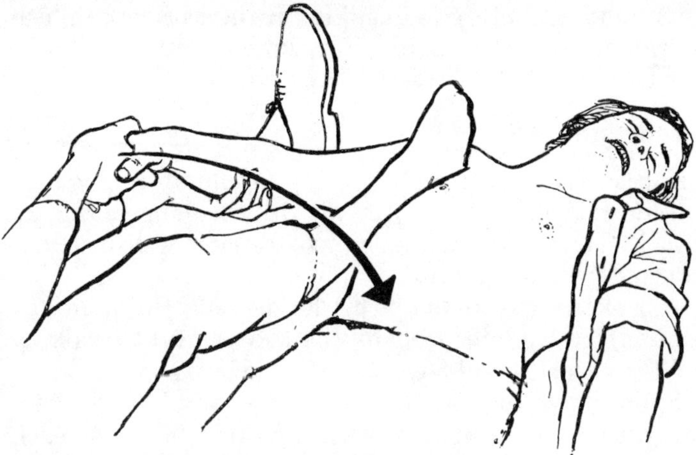

Figure 11.9 Hippocrates' shoulder reduction

— All other dislocations need only a straight pull; eschew fancy manoeuvres. So long as the splint goes on, accept a position that is less than perfect.

C. SPRAINS

When a joint is moved beyond its normal range the ligaments may be stretched or partially torn though the bones remain in their correct place. Knee cartilages are torn by twisting movements; there is much swelling and inability to straighten the leg. The signs are like a dislocation without deformity or the acute pain on movement. Firm support with a crepe bandage or elastoplast and gentle exercising is all that is required. Cold compresses of snow, bathing the limb in a cool stream and resting with the limb elevated will reduce the swelling that invariably accompanies the sprain.

It is not always easy to distinguish between a severe

sprain and a fracture (e.g. ankle). If the patient can bear weight on it then it is probably not a fracture. A simple crack fracture is best treated like a sprain anyway.

Evacuation

The casualty should walk off the mountain if possible; dallying may mean benightment with the dangers that go with it. To evacuate someone by stretcher is slow, laborious and even dangerous.

A broken arm should not hinder descent. But a broken bone in the leg will probably be too painful to walk on and the casualty will have to be carried.

Splinting should be good enough to complete the journey without continual attention to the splint. At each staging post review the condition of the casualty and his limb, to see if any modification of treatment is necessary. He may need a dressing loosened, a splint replaced or a further does of pain-killer.

12

Wounds and Poisons

A. Fresh Wounds

Most wounds can be cleaned with soap and water; dirt may have to be picked out with forceps or even scrubbed off if deeply ingrained. Immediate and thorough wound toilet will lessen the chance of infection which is bound to follow if foreign matter is left behind. The best antiseptic solution for skin cleansing is a mixture of chlorhexidine and cetrimide or either one singly.

i. Grazes, wounds and minor burns. These heal best when dry, so avoid creams which keep the skin moist and soggy. Plain paraffin gauze or gauze impregnated with antibiotic is useful for large raw areas of skin. A "non-stick" gauze dressing secured with zinc oxide plaster or sticky tape can be held in place with a conforming bandage or a crepe bandage. But these non-stick dressings often do stick, despite their name, and one of the impregnated gauzes may be better for a primary dressing. Skin abrasions heal best when left open to the air, but this may be impracticable especially if the wound is oozing blood and fluid.

ii. Small cuts. Often a small plaster dressing will suffice. If the wound edges are clean cut, close and accurate apposition will give the least final scar. This is especially important on the face.

Sterile paper strips, painless substitutes for stitches are

'butterflies' or 'dumbells' give a firmer hold. Make the surrounding skin tacky by painting with tincture of benzoin; then carefully place the strips so as to bring the very edges of the wound together and adjust the tension so it is equal all down the line.

For awkward angles — between the fingers, around the ankle — 'anchor dressings' will conform to an uneven contour. These can be easily made by cutting a piece of plaster dressing strip.

iii. Deeper wounds. Stitching stops bleeding fast, closes off the 'dead space' in the depth of the wound and holds the edges together. But you may have neither the equipment nor the skill on the mountain. Plaster or sticky tape used as shown above will suffice in emergency. Replace any skin flaps and hold skin edges accurately in position.

B. Infected Wounds

Inflammation (redness, heat and pain) mobilizes the body defences against infection; white cells in the blood gobble up germs and dead tissue forming pus.

i. Localized infection — abscess. 'Where there is pus, let it out'.

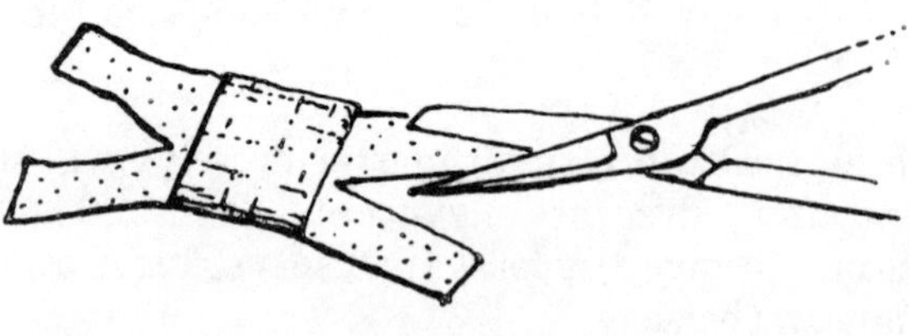

Figure 12.1 Anchor dressing

Act.

Pus will be encouraged to gather by local heat and a dressing of glycerin magnesium sulphate (GMS) paste. When 'ripe' and full of liquid pus an abscess must be lanced and kept wide open to drain. The tissue is stretched over the most prominent part so a quick stab should not be too painful, but be generous in the length of it otherwise the hole will seal over and undo the good work you have done.

Antibiotics are of use in the early stage of inflammation before pus has gathered. Local antibiotic creams are worse than useless since they may cause sensitivity to the antibiotic used.

ii. Spreading infection — cellulitis. The skin around the wound looks red and angry and feels hot and hard due to swelling. The lymph nodes draining the region (e.g. neck, armpits, groin) swell.

Act.

Immobilize the part, elevate it to reduce swelling and give antibiotics.

Poisons

a. Swallowed poisons. Most poisons swallowed accidentally or intentionally must be got rid of before they are absorbed by the blood stream.

Act.

Make the patient vomit by sticking your fingers down his throat and giving him an emetic of milk followed by a strong salty drink. A stomach washout is the most effective way of getting rid of the poison but can be dangerous if not done skilfully with a mechanical sucker at hand.

Corrosives and industrial poisons are best left lying where they are since they will burn the gullet if they are brought back up. They should be diluted by large amounts of water and/or milk.

White of egg is useful if the nature of the poison is unknown. If it was acid give toothpaste, soapsuds or washing soda; if caustic alkali give vinegar.

— Fungi. The fungi Amanita (A. phalloides = Death Cap) are easily mistaken for edible mushrooms. Avoid any 'mushrooms' that grow near trees, have white gills, a 'ring' halfway up the stalk and a remnant collar at the base.

Poisoning is manifest by violent sickness, diarrhoea and abdominal cramps coming on between 8 hours and 2 days after eating the fungi.

Act.

Stomach washouts and sedatives (diazepam).

— Deadly Nightshade (Belladonna). Atropine is the poison. The victim has widely dilated pupils and is excited, dry and flushed.

Act.

Emetics, washouts and sedatives.

b. Inhaled gas. Carbon monoxide is made by car engine combustion. In cold weather climbers sometimes camp in the back of their vans leaving the engine running to heat the inside. A small leak from the exhaust into a tightly closed space can be rapidly fatal, with little warning because the gas is odourless. When found the victim may be unconscious and very pale, and with luck, still alive.

Act.

Remove him to the fresh air, guard his airway and give assisted breathing, if possible, with oxygen. His vicious headache will need treating.

— Most camping gas is made of propane or butane and sinks to the floor. The danger of a leak is from explosion rather than poisoning.

c. *Drug abuse.* Drugs have entered the climbing scene. Unaccustomed strange behaviour, especially after a spell in camp, may be the result of a bad trip, or a 'high'. The soft drugs in common use are marihuana ('grass'), amphetamine ('speed') and LSD ('acid'). Hard drugs tend to be restricted to habitual users.

Act.

Leave purposely alone and just make sure he does not injure himself until he comes out of the trip.

13

Medical Problems

A. Heart

A 'heart attack' (coronary thrombosis) sometimes strikes out of the blue in a thirty-year-old; formerly it used to be considered an older man's illness. A warning sign of heart disease may be tightness across the chest, coming on with exertion and passing off within minutes of rest. A severe 'heart attack' is manifest by a sudden crushing pain in the centre of the chest; the pain may even start at rest, or after a meal when the patient may mistake it for indigestion. The pain can then move to the left side of the chest, down either arm, or into the neck. The victim becomes shocked and short of breath.

Act.

Rest the patient, give morphia for the pain and shock, and oxygen if he goes blue. If the heart stops start chest compression (see page 25).

B. Chest

i. Asthma. An attack of asthma is usually provoked in someone who comes in contact with a substance to which he is allergic e.g. pollen, dust, feathers, animals or certain foods. Occasionally it is due to emotional upset and is worsened by the panic of not being able to breathe. In older persons it may accompany a chest infection.

The patient becomes severely short of breath and may go blue round the lips. He wheezes because he cannot fully expel air from his lungs owing to spasm of the bronchi; this makes noisy laboured breathing.

Act.

Inhale steam from a kettle or billy-can with a towel over the head and sip hot water flavoured with lemon. One isoprenaline tablet sucked slowly or an aminophylline suppository may relax the bronchioles. If this does not help start antibiotics, and relieve anxiety with diazepam. Oxygen will help.

If the attack continues unabated and you are a long way from hospital give a steroid, preferably hydrocortisone injection or prednisone by mouth every six hours.

ii. Bronchitis and pneumonia. These two chest infections may be difficult to distinguish, but in the mountain situation their practical management is similar.

The patient has a fever, coughs hard and is short of breath. His phlegm varies from thick yellow to green and it may even be tinged with fresh or rusty blood. Breathing may hurt.

Act.

Give antibiotics in full doses for at least a week. Loosen the sputum by inhaling steam, sipping hot water with one teaspoon of baking soda and one of table salt, and thumping the chest (both sides) with the patient lying on his side with his head lower than his chest. Coughing removes infected sputum, so cough suppressants are to be discouraged. However, if sleep is impossible, codeine phosphate will dampen the cough to allow some rest. If the patient goes blue use oxygen.

iii. Spontaneous pneumothorax. Sudden pain on either side of the chest and painful shortness of breath in a young man is likely to be due to bursting of a tiny air sac in the lung with release of a little air. This will usually reabsorb over a day or two and only the pain need be treated, but the pneumothorax may cause breathlessness and warrant evacuation (see Pneumothorax, page 64).

iv. Cough fracture. After a sudden bout of hard coughing, especially at high altitudes, you may hear or feel a rib crack. Acute pain and local tenderness develop over the spot and breathing hurts.

Act.

Ease the pain and wait for healing. Injecting long-acting local anaesthetic over a rib into the fracture site makes breathing more comfortable, but take care not to slip between the ribs and puncture the lung.

C. Unconsciousness

There are several important causes, other than a simple faint or head injury, of a man found unconscious on a mountain. The victim may have a bracelet, medallion, card in his wallet or tablets in his pocket that will give a clue to a chronic condition from which he is suffering.

Act.

Whatever the cause of unconsciousness immediately turn the patient into the draining position and guard his airway.

i. Stroke. Although usually restricted to the older age groups, young persons may suffer strokes, especially as a complication of high altitude.

The patient first complains of headache, then loses consciousness. His head and eyes turn to one side and he becomes paralysed on the opposite side of the body, partially or completely. His breathing is heavy and stertorous and may have a periodic Cheyne-Stokes pattern (see page 155).

Act.

Evacuate urgently.

ii. Epilepsy. The victim lets out a sudden cry and falls to the ground. He twitches and jerks violently, his eyes roll, he froths at the mouth and may bite his tongue. The fit usually passes off in a few minutes, he wakes up and then falls into a deep sleep of recovery.

Act.

Prevent him injuring himself and put a stick between his teeth to stop him biting his tongue. Diazepam is a powerful anti-convulsant drug; a doctor can give it into a vein; if not, a muscle will do. If he is a known epileptic on treatment, make him double his dose of pills until he can have a check-up.

iii. Diabetes. Diabetics do not produce enough insulin. This hormone, or chemical messenger, controls the use of glucose in the body. Glucose is made from carbohydrates and is used as fuel to produce energy. A diabetic requires a fixed amount of carbohydrate each day and injections of insulin — given by himself — to enable him to make use of sugar. A day's climbing will entail much more exercise than usual so the diabetic is wise temporarily to increase his carbohydrate intake.

Hypoglycemia (too little sugar) occurs when a diabetic does not take enough food for his insulin to work on, or if he burns up too much sugar by exercise. Diabetic precoma (too much sugar) occurs when the patient needs more insulin or similar oral medicine. If either of these conditions gets out of control the patient is likely to slip into coma. Distinguishing between the two forms of coma is very important because the treatments are opposite.

	Hypoglycemic coma (common)	Diabetic coma (rare)
onset	sudden in a healthy person	gradual in an ill person
tongue and skin	moist	dry
breath smell	normal	acetone (acid drops)
urine taste	normal	sweet
Act:	give sugar (glucose)	give insulin

D. Jaundice

Infectious hepatitis (see page 178) is the commonest cause of jaundice that the climber is likely to meet. He feels rotten for about a week before the whites of his eyes turn yellow and his skin begins to itch.

Several infectious diseases especially those caused by viruses have this preliminary stage of malaise before the illness becomes obvious e.g. influenza, glandular fever, pharyngitis but there is no jaundice.

Act.

Rest and get medical advice. Avoid alcohol.

PSYCHOLOGICAL PROBLEMS

Most people's psychological problems are fortunately alleviated by the peace of the hills. For this very reason many of us choose them as our escape from worldly cares.

We must be able to distinguish panic from psychosis.

a. Panic. Under arduous mountain conditions or during a difficult ascent the climber may lose his nerve and become frightened, agitated and acutely anxious. Although he remains rational he is paralysed with fear so that he becomes totally ineffectual.

Act.

Talk him down with calm reassurance; anger will only provoke him. When he is back at camp sedate him heavily with diazepam. Wait until next morning to see if he comes back to normal after he has slept off the drug; if he does it is the surest distinction between panic and psychosis. He will probably be deeply ashamed of the episode, so avoid mention of it unless he wishes to talk to get it off his chest. Remember that such emotions might be the lot of any of us.

b. Psychosis. Madness, as distinct from panic, does not usually start out of the blue without some previous warning that the person was unbalanced mentally. In selecting a climbing team be cautious of someone with a record of strange behaviour.

The patient may lose touch with reality and have bizarre hallucinations. He feels that other people are ganging up on him and he may appear so convincing that you begin to wonder who is sick, you or he. He tends to over-react to normal situations and may be violent and excited, or passive and withdrawn.

After the acute phase of a psychotic episode a more drawn-out depression sets in; this is the time the patient is most likely to try to kill himself.

Act.

Heavy sedation with diazepam will be needed to quieten him and if he becomes violent try to prevent him from injuring himself and others. Forcibly restraining him may only make him more excited, but may be needed in the last resort.

14

Surgical Emergencies

The following conditions will ultimately, and some of them urgently, warrant the attention, though not necessarily the knife, of a surgeon. Acute bellyache may be encountered in any group of fit climbers; once you have excluded constipation, and the gripes of a simple tummy upset due to gluttony or careless living, the most likely serious cause is acute appendicitis.

A. Appendicitis

Appendicitis can be a very easy diagnosis to make when all the classical signs are present, and yet in its early stages it can be the most difficult as it is easily confused with so many other conditions. The signs vary widely not only with the stage of the disease but with the position where the very mobile appendix is lying. It is an organ about the size of a finger attached to the caecum, which is the start of the large bowel, lying in the right lower quarter of the abdomen. The reason for giving so much space to appendicitis is because it can be very serious if not dealt with and surgery is *the* treatment, so the only place for a suspected case is hospital – pronto.

Ask.

Commonly the person complains of discomfort starting round the umbilicus; the pain then shifts to the right lower quarter of the abdomen. Food is revolting, he feels queasy, is usually constipated and may vomit *after* the onset of pain (vomiting is not a feature of 'women's problems' see section 5). Walking may hurt in the right groin only.

Look.

The temperature and pulse are usually raised, the furred tongue is a dirty brown and the breath is foul. A scar over the tender point may show that the appendix has already been snatched.

Feel.

Gently press on the patient's abdomen with a flat hand and the muscles on the right side will tense as he 'guards' the tender contents of his belly, whereas the left side remains soft. Pressing more deeply in the right lower quarter almost invariably makes him say 'Ouch!'

Act.

The danger of appendicitis is that the inflamed appendix can burst within hours of onset of the illness, spilling pus into the belly and causing peritonitis which may be lethal.

If there is no way of reaching hospital soon, it is reasonable to treat the patient with double doses of a broad-spectrum antibiotic in the hope of dampening the infection. Meantime allow only sips of water, place a soothing hot water bottle on his abdomen and be generous with the pain-killers.

The most common conditions that may mimic appendicitis, roughly in order of occurrence, are:

1. *Constipation.* A suggestive story of constipation may be proved by a laxative suppository — safer than pills because it is less violent.

2. *Kidney infection (pyelitis).* The patient passes urine

frequently and it is cloudy or even blood-tinged, feels tender in the loin, will have a high fever and may suffer shaking rigors. This condition is far commoner in females than males.

Act.

Drink gallons and take a broad-spectrum antibiotic.

3. *Kidney stone.* Agonizing colic occurs when a small stone passes down the ureter, the tube that connects the kidney to the bladder. The patient tends to roll around with pain, which starts in the loin and moves towards the groin; it comes in waves, builds up to a crescendo when the victim may vomit; then the pain dies down leaving a dull ache. Water is passed frequently and may be blood-stained. Stones are encouraged to form by dehydration.

Act.

Drink heavily (water), take strong pain-killers and pray while waiting for the inevitable passing of the stone.

4. *Acute gall-bladder (cholecystitis).* Constant pain is usually felt high under the right ribs; it travels through to the back or up into the right shoulder blade. The whites of the eyes may turn yellow-jaundiced and food is nauseating.

Act.

Antibiotics may quieten the attack.

5. *Women's problems.* Abandon prudery and ask any woman complaining of low bellyache the date of her last period and whether she might be pregnant.

— If she is expecting a period the pain may be the normal premenstrual 'curse' pains which can, however, be extremely disabling. If the date is exactly halfway between her periods an egg may be rupturing from her ovary giving acute pain and lingering tenderness, which usually passes off after a few hours.

Act.

Give sympathy and mild pain-killers.

— If she may be pregnant — beware of:—

i. Abortion (miscarriage). The story of a missed period with heavy bleeding and generalized cramping pains is suggestive.

ii. Ectopic pregnancy. Rarely a pregnancy develops outside the womb in one or other uterine tube. An early ectopic in the right tube may mimic appendicitis and it can suddenly burst out and cause profuse bleeding into the belly. If in doubt tip the patient head down and if she gets pain in the shoulders it suggests blood has trickled up under the diaphragm and is irritating the phrenic nerve.

Act.

Get the lady to hospital quickly.

6. Perforated peptic ulcer (see next paragraph).

B. Peptic Ulcer

Ulcers in the stomach or duodenum may exist for years without causing more trouble than vague indigestion and discomfort in the pit of the stomach. They can be controlled by avoiding fats, drinking milk and taking antacid tablets. But if an ulcer bleeds or perforates the ensuing crisis may be sudden and catastrophic; in both cases the urgent attention of a surgeon is needed.

i. Bleeding. The patient feels faint and sweaty, vomits bright red or coffee ground blood (haematemesis) and quickly becomes shocked. He may have diarrhoea some hours later with dark tarry stools.

ii. Perforation. Pain in the upper abdomen, so severe that you mistake it for a heart attack, starts suddenly. Peritonitis sets in as spilled stomach contents and bacteria spread throughout the abdominal cavity and pain gets steadily worse all over the belly. The patient vomits and his pulse rises. When the initial shock subsides he may appear to improve, but this deceptive phase precedes collapse. The tender abdomen becomes rigid as a plank and his breathing is shallow and he looks, and is, deathly.

Act.

In both cases treat the shock and start antibiotics.

C. Hernia (Rupture)

A hernia is a swelling in the groin that may contain gut and protrudes through the muscular wall of the abdomen into the groin, and may be nothing more than an inconvenience. It may slide back on lying down, either by itself or with the help of gentle pressure. The danger of a hernia is that it may be nipped off causing obstruction of the bowel. If this is not relieved the bowel becomes strangulated, turns gangrenous and perforates. The patient will have a tense tender swelling in the groin that cannot be pushed back; he may develop forcible vomiting, griping pains and a distended abdomen.

Act.

Rest the patient with his feet up and head down to encourage the hernia to slide back into the abdomen on its own accord. Give big doses of an analgesic and flex his hips to help the muscles relax and so allow you to gently squeeze the hernia back. If it does not go easily, do not force it; flee to hospital.

D. Testicle

If a testicle becomes inflamed or is kicked it swells and is exquisitely tender. Sudden pain *without* a story of injury is likely to be due to twisting which must be dealt with urgently by a surgeon.

Act.

Support the scrotum in a tight pair of pants well padded with cotton-wool, start antibiotics and don't make the patient laugh.

E. Haemorrhoids (Piles)

Mountaineers are prone to piles, especially at high altitudes, probably because of carrying unaccustomed heavy loads. They are varicose veins of the anus and are uncomfortable and inconvenient. Any suspicion of piles warrants the needle of a surgeon to shrivel them up before they give trouble. Commonly a speck of bright blood appears on the toilet paper after passing a hard stool and there may be a maddening itch and slimy discharge.

Act.

Avoid constipation and use a haemorrhoidal cream or suppository.

If piles prolapse from the anus push them back immediately by hand because the longer they remain out the more difficult it will be to make them go back. Dropping your trousers at 20,000 ft. in a blizzard for your 'daily' is bad enough, but to have prolapsed piles as well constitutes the sum total of human misery.

F. Toothache

Toothache can be so disabling and cause sufficient pain and malaise as to render the climber a useless member of his party. Intense cold, especially at high altitude makes diseased or exposed teeth painful, and when cold teeth are suddenly warmed by a hot drink or biting on hard food they tend to fracture.

Most toothache can be prevented by a careful dental check including X-rays before setting off, a diet with adequate vitamin C during the expedition and continued hygiene by regularly cleaning your teeth. Rubbing the teeth with a wet finger covered with salt or a peeled green stick is a good substitute for a toothbrush. Chewing gum keeps the mouth clean and exercises the gums.

The causes of toothache are legion but have been pruned here for simplicity. Dental pain has many guises:- aching, throbbing, searing — and may be difficult to localize to a particular tooth, especially in the early stages. Pain often affects adjacent teeth and may spread from the upper to the lower jaw and vice-versa, but never across the mid-line.

Localization of an Aching Tooth

i. Knocking. Knock the suspected tooth on the top and side with the handle of a metal dental probe. This will cause pain if it is diseased.

ii. Probing. Stick the point of the probe into the exposed cavity or the softened exposed root.

iii. Cooling. Cold worsens the pain in living teeth; heat does the same in dead ones.

Pain from an infected maxillary sinus (the air space behind the cheek) can mimic pain in the upper jaw and is a common reason for faulty extraction of healthy teeth. In sinusitis, knocking or pressing the cheek of the patient with a finger produces pain, there may be a snotty discharge from the nose, and if pain is on both sides it is unlikely to be due to a bad tooth.

An amateur in the field is limited to giving very simple treatment to tide the patient over until he can see a proper dentist.

Common Causes of Toothache

1. Abscess. An abscess forms round the root of a decaying tooth. The throbbing pain is partly relieved by clenching the jaw and then opening the mouth. The face and jaw swell, the breath smells foul and pain is severe.

Act.

— Antibiotics. Penicillin or one of its broad-spectrum relatives (ampicillin) is the drug of choice.

— Pain-killers. Analgesics may be able to deal with the milder sorts of pain. Oil of cloves put onto the tooth or into the cavity may give temporary relief; hot salt mouthwashes are soothing, cleansing and encourage pus to discharge into the mouth.

If this treatment fails, pain continues and adjacent teeth become involved the tooth may have to be extracted (see below).

2. Cavities. A breach in the enamel due to decay, a lost filling or a fractured tooth lays bare the sensitive inner dentine layer or the actual pulp or "nerve" of the tooth which is very painful.

Act.

A temporary dressing can be made from zinc oxide powder mixed with oil of cloves, or a synthetic cement ('Cavit') that comes in a tiny tube and does not harden so long as it is stoppered. The paste is pushed into the hole with a finger and pressed down with any tool or a matchstick. A dental probe is useful for digging out the remnants of fillings.

3. *Exposed tooth root.* When open to the cold exposed roots cause much pain which may develop into chronic toothache if not dealt with.

Act.

'Tresiolan' or even 'Sensodyne' toothpaste rubbed into the area relieve pain. Avoid heavy tooth brushing.

4. *Gum infections (severe).* The gums swell painfully, ulcerate and bleed causing an evil odour. Unerupted wisdom teeth are particularly susceptible.

Act.

Careful and efficient toothbrushing is essential. Gentian violet paint, made up from crystals, is good for dealing with most sorts of mouth ulcers though it is very messy to use. The antibiotic to use is metronidazole.

Extraction

The art of extracting a loose or bad tooth can be learnt easily enough, but to remove a strong live tooth is very difficult. You need the proper tools and a stoical patient as you will probably not have the expertise to use a local anaesthetic. Unskilled needle-jabbing in the mouth will be very painful and is unlikely to be effective. Several swigs of neat alcohol and a strong pain-killer is a good alternative.

With a pair of 'upper' or 'lower' dental forceps grasp the appropriate tooth close to the gum margin, pushing the beaks down each side to below gum level in order to get as far down the root as possible. Then using a sideways rocking and rotating movement try to work the tooth loose. Do not be put off by the crunching noise that comes from the jaw as the roots separate from the socket. If the tooth breaks try to grasp and remove the remaining fragments but do not go digging deeply for them or you may start profuse bleeding. Squeeze the gums together with a finger pinch to stop bleeding from the socket and get the patient to bite on a damp gauze pack or handkerchief for 15 minutes. If you can stop the bleeding in no other way, pack the socket with gauze. Even removing the tooth crown alone may diminish the pain by letting pus discharge down the roots into the mouth. Do not allow the patient to smoke on the same day as this may restart bleeding. Start hot salt mouthwashes on the second day.

15

Eyes, Ears, Nose and Throat

EYES

The eyeball holds a special horror for many people and few can bring themselves to inspect it closely let alone touch it.

Look.

Examine the patient's eyes with a strong torch beam and a magnifying glass (a camera lens held close to your own eye).

Pull down the lower lid to look for foreign bodies in the lower gutter and then evert the upper lid as this is a common place for uninvited matter to lodge. Inspect the lid margins closely for inturned lashes which scratch the cornea and are the source of much hidden discomfort.

Redness of the conjunctiva (the loose membrane over the white sclera of the eye) denotes inflammation or infection, which may cause aversion to bright light and tears or even pussy discharge. The cornea (window of the eye) should normally be clear, shiny and even. Any breach in its surface will show up as a bright green stain when a paper strip impregnated with fluorescein is touched against the damp inner lid. The stain spreads around the eye so abrasions, ulcers and foreign bodies are more easily seen. The pupil is normally circular and becomes smaller when light is shone into it; an eccentric pupil suggests something is wrong in the front chamber of the eye.

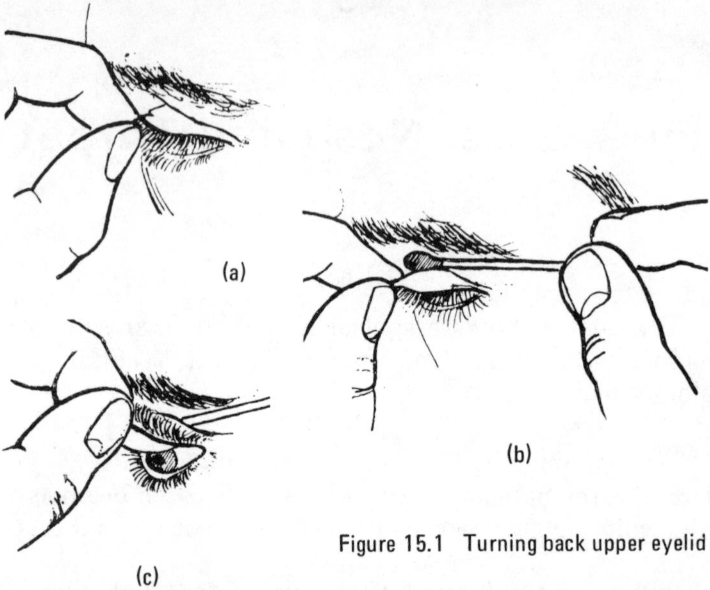

Figure 15.1 Turning back upper eyelid

By testing the vision you can roughly assess the state of the eye, which is all you can do without an ophthalmoscope (an instrument for looking into the back of the eye) and the skill to use it. Ask the casualty to read, with glasses if he normally uses them, newsprint of various sizes from a normal reading distance. Test each eye singly and ask if each was in full working order before the injury. Recording the vision now will help comparison later.

Act.

Emergency care of most eye conditions will have to be kept simple until the casualty can be seen by a specialist.

— Cover. Most inflamed or injured eyes abhor strong light. If one eye only is affected hold an eye pad (or a gauze square) in place with sticky tape; if both eyes, use dark glasses. A firm bandage over the pad gives added comfort.

— Drugs. Ointments are generally more use than drops as they stay around the eye for longer and need only be put in once or twice a day.

a. Antibiotics. Chloramphenicol gives the broadest protection; neomycin and sulphacetamide are alternatives. Antiseptics have little place and patent remedies containing mercury (golden eye ointment) may cause dangerous sensitivity reactions.

b. Steroids. Hydrocortisone and prednisolone have a magical effect on many red eyes but are best avoided unless in skilled hands as, in the presence of herpes virus infection, they can be dangerous.

c. Pupil dilators. Homatropine dilates the pupil and relieves painful spasm that comes on after injury; it temporarily blurs the vision and makes the eye sensitive to light so dark glasses or a cover are necessary. Homatropine is short-acting, needs to be put in twice a day, and the danger of inducing glaucoma is negligible. Atropine may leave the pupil dilated for a couple of weeks.

d. Local anaesthetics. Amethocaine removes all feeling from the sensitive cornea so it can be touched and foreign bodies can be removed. But the eye must always be covered afterwards until its natural protective sensation returns.

Common Eye Problems

A. Painful Red Eye

i. Conjunctivitis. Both eyes feel gritty as though there is sand in them; they look red, may water or discharge and resent bright light. If one single eye is affected and the vision blurred, inflammation of the iris or a foreign body is more likely.

Act.

Use dark glasses and antibiotic ointment.

ii. Foreign body. A speck of dirt or metal is seen embedded in the cornea or conjunctiva or hidden in the fornices.

Act.

Wash the eye with ample water. Try to wipe the speck away with the dampened corner of a handkerchief or a wisp of cotton wool wound onto a match stick. If it will not budge, anaesthetise the eye and cautiously scrape the speck off with a sterile needle. Refrain if it does not come away easily. Then treat as a corneal abrasion.

iii. Corneal abrasion. A minute breach in the surface of the cornea is very painful. Abrasions can be caused by inturned lashes, walking into twigs or pine needles and splinters from chopping wood. Ulcers follow infection.

Act.

If an eyelash offends thee, pluck it out; if a foreign body, remove it. Then dilate the pupil, apply antibiotic ointment and cover the eye with a pad and bandage. Most abrasions heal within 24–48 hours. Corneal ulcers take much longer but basically need the same treatment.

iv. Burns. When the face is burned the lids take the brunt of the damage as they usually close before flame touches the cornea. Corneal burns occur from fire sparks, chemicals and ultraviolet light (snow-blindness).

Act.

Wash the eye copiously with water; better still, use bicarbonate of soda against acids or milk for caustic alkaline burns.

B. Globe Injury

i. Bruising. A small blow or even rubbing the eyes during sleep can cause a drop of blood to spread under the conjunctiva. A horrifying bright red eye appears but it is of no sinister importance and needs no treatment; the colour fades in several days.

Serious bruising of the eye always affects the sight either by causing general dimness or blank patches in the field of vision. Blood may appear in the chamber behind the cornea in front of the pupil, inside the eyeball, or the retina may become detached.

Act.

Rest the eye by covering it and seek help urgently.

ii. Penetration. Fluid may be spilled from the anterior chamber making an irregular pupil. The iris lies close up against the cornea or even is pinched in the wound. As in 'open' fractures of bones, infection is the greatest hazard.

The opposite uninjured eye is always at risk after a penetrating injury because of 'sympathetic' inflammation which can quickly lead to blindness.

Act.

Dilate the pupil, use antibiotic ointment, pad and bandage and give antibiotics by mouth.

Seek help urgently.

C. Eyelid Injury

Poor healing of lids may cause serious problems with their delicate windscreen-wiper mechanism. Expert surgery is needed for their repair.

EARS

i. Acute earache (otitis media). A searing pain develops in the affected ear, with fever.

Act.

Give large doses of penicillin. A light cotton wool plug in the ear opening keeps out cold and reduces pain, which will need strong treatment. Drops or powder do good only for otitis externa when there is a smelly discharge from the outer ear but little pain.

ii. Foreign body. Lumps of wax, round objects the size of beans, and insects occasionally get into the outer ear.

Act.

Lubricate the passage with liquid paraffin. Turn the head on one side and shake vigorously. Then syringe the ear with warm water to help the object slide out. Do not poke around with matchsticks or the ear drum may be damaged.

NOSE

i. Nosebleeds. This minor annoyance usually stops on its own after a few minutes, but it may be so severe and uncontrollable as to threaten life. It is never a 'safety valve'. Bleeding usually arises from the septum between the nostrils or high in the nose, well out of sight.

Act.

Sit the patient up, leaning slightly forward with his head bowed. Encourage him to blow out of his nostrils clots, which do nothing to stop further bleeding and just dam up behind them blood that trickles down the back of the throat instead. Swallowed blood will make him vomit. Look carefully to see from which side the blood is coming and try to identify the actual spot. Place a cold compress, preferably using ice or snow, across the bridge of his nose.

Squeeze the nostrils together high up where the bone and soft nose cartilage join, and make the patient bite on a stick to prevent him swallowing, yet permit mouth breathing. If bleeding still does not stop push a gauze pack as high as possible to plug the offending nostril and leave it in place for 24–48 hours. The mountainside is no place for trying to pack the post-nasal space via the mouth — a manoeuvre fraught with hazard.

ii. Broken nose. This unimportant fracture may mar your beauty. When the swelling has subsided a surgeon can consider straightening it.

THROAT

i. Sore throat.

a. Virus infections are a common cause. The throat looks fiery red, there is no pus but the infection does not respond to antibiotics.

Act.

Gargle with aspirin dissolved in warm water and then swallow the gargle; this provides better relief than most fancy medicines.

b. Breathing the cold dry air of high mountains causes a raw dry throat.

Act.

Inhale steam from a bowl or sniff a billy can on the stove while making a tea brew to moisten the air, but don't scald your nose or throat in the process. Cough sweets soothe but are always in short supply.

ii. Tonsillitis. Yellow flecks of pus lie on the red and swollen tonsils, and glands in the neck swell. Swallowing is painful and difficult.

Act.

Penicillin and aspirin gargles.

iii. Glandular fever. If the above treatment for 'tonsillitis' has no effect on a throat with a thick yellow slough that looks far worse than it feels, suspect glandular fever. You feel rotten for a couple of weeks, and rest is the best cure. If the throat becomes so swollen that swallowing and breathing are seriously impaired take a course of prednisone, for five days.

iv. Quinsy. An abscess develops in the region of the tonsil bed, the soft palate swells and swallowing may be almost impossible.

Act.

Urgent decisive lancing into the upper pole of the affected tonsil should release a gush of pus. Follow this with warm salt water or aspirin gargles and penicillin.

v. Swallowed foreign body. Fishbones stuck in the gullet

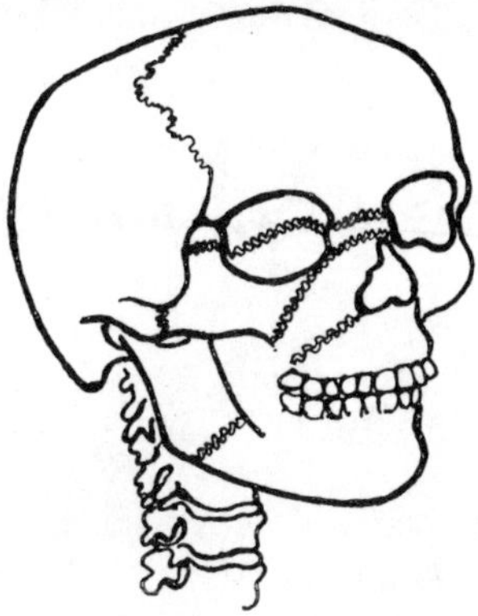

Figure 15.2 Face and jaw fracture sites

can often be dislodged by eating dry bread. An unmovable bone will have to be taken to a surgeon.

FACE AND JAWS

The facial bones may be broken in several places in a badly smashed face. Suspect such fractures if the bite does not bring the teeth together normally or if the patient has double vision, a bruised cheek and black eye, and if you can feel a step in the line of his lower eye socket bone.

Broken jaw and face bones need expert treatment urgently.

16

Altitude Acclimatization

ACCLIMATIZATION

Man learns to live and work in the oxygen-depleted atmosphere of high altitudes by acclimatization. The air we breathe at sea-level is composed of four parts of nitrogen and one part of oxygen (20%). As we climb higher and higher the 4:1 ratio of these gases does not change but their density becomes less and the pressure exerted by them falls steadily. An ordinary weather barometer registers the pressure that gases in the atmosphere exert on the surface of the earth and can therefore be used as an altimeter. At the top of Mt. Blanc (15,780 ft., 4,800 m.) the oxygen pressure is just over half that at sea-level; on the summit of Mount Everest (29,002 ft., 8,848 m.) it is less than one third.

A time will come when the steadily diminishing pressure is no longer adequate to drive sufficient oxygen into the tissues. Oxygen is essential for the life and function of all the cells in the body, and the more sensitive the cell the greater its demand for oxygen. If deprived of oxygen, brain cells die in less than four minutes.

If the body made no adjustments to compensate for the low pressure of oxygen life would be unendurable above about 10,000 ft. (3,000 m.). High altitude mountaineering is only possible because the physiological changes involved in acclimatization are ultimately directed to one end: keeping the body adequately supplied with oxygen.

The initial rapid phase of acclimatization starts at about 5,000 ft. (1,500 m.) when the low oxygen pressure in the atmosphere, and hence in the lungs and the blood, is detected by small chemical receptor organs placed in the carotid arteries on the way to the brain.

1. Breathing

At sea level the rate and depth of breathing are controlled by the level of carbon dioxide waste produced by the body tissues. At about, or over, 10,000 ft. (3,000 m.) this normally sensitive carbon dioxide control is overridden by the paramount need to get enough oxygen. Lack of oxygen increases the rate and depth of breathing so carbon dioxide levels in the blood fall briskly until a steady state for that individual at that altitude is reached.

Breathing increases because the carotid chemical receptors send nervous impulses to stimulate the respiratory centre in the brain. With deeper breathing carbon dioxide, which dilutes oxygen in the lungs, is removed more rapidly and its concentration in the blood falls. This has the effect of dampening the activity of the respiratory centre, so we end up with a delicate balance between two opposing forces — a low oxygen and a low carbon dioxide pressure — controlling the rate and depth of breathing.

— Cheyne-Stokes, or periodic breathing.

A change in breathing rhythm is common on arrival at altitude and is particularly noticeable and worrying at night. Breathing gradually grows deeper rising to a peak; it then falls off and finally ceases completely for several seconds so the person may wake up and think he is dying. Then this alarming pattern starts all over again.

The reason for Cheyne-Stokes breathing is not understood. The carbon dioxide in the blood builds up and when it reaches a sufficient concentration the respiratory centre, abnormally responsive to oxygen lack like a too-sensitive thermostat, is stimulated and breathing restarts. Carbon dioxide is then blown off by breathing, the stimulus lessens and breathing comes to a standstill. With acclimatization this abnormal behaviour of the respiratory centre ceases and it settles down to a new level of stimulation by carbon dioxide.

2. Heart

The heart beats faster and more strongly, noticed as palpitations in the chest and a dull 'sinus' headache beating in time with the pulse.

The low oxygen pressure stimulates both the carotid chemical receptors and the sympathetic nervous system to make the heart work as a more efficient pump. It pushes a greater volume of blood to the lungs each minute and therefore more oxygen becomes available to the tissues where it is readily released because of the relative differences in pressure between the blood and the tissues. Many tiny capillaries open up so that every cell has more blood available, and oxygen is delivered, and carbon dioxide removed, more efficiently.

Other symptoms noticed early on are difficulty in sleeping and a nasal quality in the speech. Now the *slower phase of acclimatization* takes over.

3. Blood and Plasma

Soon after arriving at altitude the volume of plasma, the fluid in which the blood cells are suspended, is diminished by 20-30%; this is partly because more urine is passed as you climb, partly because you become dehydrated by sweating with heavy exercise and overbreathing in the cold dry atmosphere, which causes evaporation. Water losses are hard to replenish above the snow line because snow has to be melted to meet the normal daily requirement of 3–4 litres.

New blood cells are made in the bone marrow which is stimulated by the low oxygen pressure to produce more red cells, but this may take 4–6 weeks to be fully effective. There is, as a result, more haemoglobin available to carry more oxygen. At high altitude blood can carry up to half as much oxygen again as at sea-level.

As the red cells increase and the plasma diminishes, the blood becomes thicker or more viscous. The heart is put under strain pumping sticky fluid round the body, and the circulation slows. Red cells tend to clump together forming thromboses, a tendency that is increased when men have to 'fester' in their tents during long periods of bad weather, because the leg muscles are inefficient at pumping blood in the leg veins back to the heart. Small blood clots may break off and lodge in the fine vessels of the lung or brain. Mild 'strokes' have been recorded on several Himalayan expeditions.

4. Miscellaneous

Changes occur in the body chemistry, myoglobin of muscle and the enzyme systems, with one end in view — to make the most use of what little oxygen is available in the thin air on high.

All these facts indicate that various parts of the acclimatization process start at different levels of altitude and proceed at different rates, and this process may be entirely painless and pass almost unnoticed. Some people are never troubled by the height provided they ascend slowly enough, while others for no obvious physical reason can never acclimatize properly however long they remain high, even if this height is comparatively modest. This feature of altitude is very individual and idiosyncratic.

Ironically acclimatization is not always a continuing process. Deterioration can start after about three months at very high altitude, say above 19,000 ft. (6,000m.), and gets steadily worse. You do not work or sleep well, you lose appetite and weight. The only answer is retreat to the valleys for a long rest.

ACUTE MOUNTAIN SICKNESS

Acute mountain sickness is the most traditional and simple term for what befalls those who fail to acclimatize. Anyone venturing above 10–12,000 ft. (3,000–3,600 m.) is wise to learn something about this insidious illness which can be rapidly fatal if not recognized and treated promptly.

Most people who climb high are fit on arrival but then feel ghastly for a day or two, with severe lassitude, frontal headaches, nausea, vomiting, loss of appetite and sleeplessness. These symptoms, which are due to a little water on the brain, tend to pass off as they acclimatize. But a few never get used to the altitude and may become seriously ill.

How?

At high altitudes surplus body water is normally shed by passing more urine. However in certain susceptible and quite unpredictable people, water is retained in the body and settles in the wrong places — on the lungs (High Altitude Pulmonary Oedema, HAPE) or in the cells of the brain (High Altitude Cerebral Oedema, HACE). The precise cause of Acute Mountain Sickness is unknown and whether the mechanics of these two syndromes is similar is still uncertain.

All the early signs of Acute Mountain Sickness can be explained by water accumulating in the brain cells which lose the ability to keep water out because they are deprived of oxygen. The brain swells inside its rigid box, the skull, the cerebral blood vessels dilate and the flow of blood through them increases, so the overall effect is that the pressure of cerebro-spinal fluid rises. The swollen brain has nowhere to expand, so it presses on nerve centres at the base of the brain. The vital functions they control, like breathing and heart rate, are upset.

It is impossible to predict who will suffer from Acute Mountain Sickness, or when. Previous acclimatization helps but fitness and training guarantee no protection, and no age is exempt. Cold, fear, dehydration, fatigue and taking heavy exercise soon after rapid ascent predispose to the illness. Slow and steady acclimatization, taking plenty of time over the ascent, reduces the chances of getting Acute Mountain Sickness, which does not usually come on until 2–3 days after arrival. Those who have suffered before are likely to suffer again.

It is no disgrace to take the approach at a very gentle and leisurely pace; Odell, Shipton and Whillans always have done. The secret is not to climb too high too fast; and when you are up, carry high but sleep low.

Look.

Beware of the climber who does not acclimatize well and is feeling, and going, less well than you would expect for the height and his previous performance. The stiff-upper-lip tough guy who battles ever upward in the face of increasing distress is the one most likely to end up under a cairn of stones with a wooden cross on top.

The victim feels sick and complains that his head aches and feels tight as if blown up like a balloon. His face appears puffy and hands are swollen so that rings may feel tight. He may notice that he passes markedly less urine than normal.

HIGH ALTITUDE CEREBRAL OEDEMA

Fortunately this is rare. The brain bulges when a lot of water collects and many tiny haemorrhages are scattered in it. Throbbing headache, like a severe migraine, is the predominant symptom. The climber is apathetic and irrational, staggers as if drunk, and sees double; he may then have a fit and sink into coma.

Retinal Haemorrhages

Looking at the vessels of the retina in the back of the eye with an ophthalmoscope gives a good idea what is happening in the vessels of the brain. One in every three climbers going above 20,000 ft. (6,000 m.), and possibly even at lower altitudes, will have marked changes in the retina. The blood vessels become fat and tortuous and much more blood flows through them. They tend to burst, possibly because the huge pressures developed in the chest on coughing are transmitted to the brain, and flame-shaped haemorrhages are seen scattered throughout the background of the eye. The head of the optic nerve may be swollen suggesting pressure inside the skull.

The climber may complain of spots before the eyes, or blank patches in his field of vision or he may not notice anything abnormal.

HIGH ALTITUDE PULMONARY OEDEMA

The lung is water-logged so oxygen has difficulty in passing across from the alveoli to the blood. The oedema is caused partly by blocked and leaking capillaries, and partly because the vessels are narrowed yet trying to cope with an overloaded lung circulation. There is no sign of heart failure.

The victim is short of breath, hungry for air, and looks blue round the lips; his chest crackles loudly and his sputum appears frothy and pink or blood-stained.

Act.

a. Descent. For both conditions urgent and immediate descent to a lower altitude is vital and often miraculous; this is one of the few truly substantiated facts in a subject shrouded in speculation. A patient near death from pulmonary oedema at Everest Base Camp can be quite normal on arrival at Kathmandu after an hour's helicopter flight. Taking someone down even 3,000 ft. (1,000 m.), or preferably lower, can make a noticeable difference. However, sufferers from cerebral oedema can remain unconscious for days and yet recover completely.

Other forms of treatment play for time but should never take preference over immediately evacuating the patient to a lower altitude, even if it is in the middle of the night. Drugs and oxygen may tide the patient over but must not delude you into delay.

b. Rest. Rest the casualty propped up, so oedema fluid sinks to the bottom of his lungs and pools in his legs. Keep him warm and relaxed because cold and anxiety aggravate the illness.

c. Oxygen. Oxygen helps to relieve panting and change the patient's blue colour to pink, but do not be deceived by his apparent, temporary improvement. He still needs to be evacuated urgently.

d. Drugs.

— Diuretics. These help the patient to pass urine and so to shed some of the body water that has accumulated in the wrong places (brain and lung).

i. Acetazolamide ('Diamox') is a mild diuretic, and has some effect in preventing the onset of oedema especially of the brain, in a susceptible person if taken 2–3 days before and 2–3 days after arrival at, but not throughout, the stay at altitude. Do not rely on this drug to prevent Acute Mountain Sickness.

ii. Frusemide ('Lasix') has a powerful diuretic effect on someone who has definite High Altitude Pulmonary Oedema, but it severely depletes the body water and so must not be used routinely for prevention, as dehydration contributes to the cause of Acute Mountain Sickness. For this reason you must encourage the patient to drink especially if the diuretics are working well.

— Steroids. Beta- or dexamethasone, preferably injected, are helpful in treating cerebral oedema, but do not start to act for at least 6 hours.

— Morphine. In pulmonary oedema morphine allays anxiety, encourages urine flow, shifts blood away from the lungs, and so eases breathing. But it must be given with great caution as the drug can severely depress breathing. It must not be used in cerebral oedema.

With good sense Acute Mountain Sickness and its sinister offspring, High Altitude Pulmonary and Cerebral Oedema, should not happen; if they do so rapid evacuation to a lower altitude should prevent their deadly consequences.

17

Frostbite

Frostbite is rare among skilled mountaineers and people used to living in Arctic and Antarctic climates, who avoid trouble by wearing protective clothing and by being constantly aware of the dangers of cold. Tibetans, Andean Indians and Eskimos adapt to their cold and hostile environment by knowing how to survive and how to look after themselves by their own intuitive cunning. Longstanding weathering of their hands and faces makes them appear to have some inborn defence against cold, but they can suffer its ravages like the rest of us.

Cold is determined by the combined effect of air temperature and wind speed; this is known as 'windchill'. In still air and sunshine with a temperature of − 40°C you can walk about in shirt sleeves and feel comfortably warm, but when the wind speed rises to 30 or 40 m.p.h. the cold at even − 1°C may be intolerable. At these temperatures wet cold is unusual as snow falls instead of rain.

Frostbite results from freezing of the tissues, which then become injured and may die. Hands and feet are commonly frostbitten because blood has to travel so far to reach and warm them and their large surface area allows them to lose heat rapidly. Faces, noses and ears may be nipped if they are inadequately protected. Frostbite cools the surface tissues, in contrast to exposure (hypothermia) in which the temperature of the deep inner core of the body falls (see Chapter 15). If the core temperature remains normal the extremities have less chance of freezing.

In severe cold weather at any altitude, frostbite is an ever-present hazard which becomes a reality when an accident happens. The victim may be immobilized because of pain and unable to increase his body heat by exercise. When unconscious, the shivering reflex, one of the most important inborn ways of heat production, may even be abolished. Fear associated with the accident causes emotional shock and blood vessels in the extremities of the body clamp down so the limbs become cold; loss of blood from a wound or into a fracture site can produce clinical shock. Any open wound in which tissue is damaged is readily frostbitten.

The risk of frostbite increases the higher you climb because the air temperature falls and the wind makes the effect of cold more severe. At really high altitudes – over about 20,000 ft. (6,000 m.) fatigue is excessive because of the greater physical effort needed to work in an oxygen depleted atmosphere and difficulty in sleeping. The brain becomes dulled and you tend to become careless about normal self-defence against hostile surroundings. On Annapurna in 1958 Herzog dropped his gloves but forgot that he carried in his rucksack a pair of socks which he could have used as mittens and so prevented some of the terrible injury he suffered.

At great heights food is boring, appetite is poor and it is difficult to melt enough snow for drinking-water because fuel is scarce. Red blood cells multiply in order to carry more oxygen, so the blood is thicker and more viscous and flows sluggishly. Small clots tend to form in the vessels because climbers often have to lie 'festering' in their tents in bad weather for days at a time not taking the exercise that is needed to stimulate their circulation.

Frost will 'bite' the unwary causing devastating disability and even death. So take good care to avoid it.

PRECAUTIONS

Clothing

a. Body. Windproof clothing is essential; it must also be waterproof at lower altitudes where rain falls instead of snow. When air is displaced by wind or wet, insulation fails.

b. Face. The face is easily frostbitten because it is difficult to cover completely; ears and noses cool quickly because they project from the face and have a large surface area. Wear a balaclava helmet or wool hat that leaves only a small opening for the middle of the face; a silk scarf tied over the mouth and nose still allows you to breathe comfortably and is also excellent protection against the glare of the sun that burns lips and noses. Keep an eye open for white blanched areas on the faces of your companions and take action quickly if they appear.

c. Hands. Hands must be covered yet still able to handle rope, ice-axe and camera. Mittens allow the fingers to move freely and to warm each other by contact whereas gloves isolate each finger and may constrict the circulation. If you have to perform delicate manual tasks or to handle cold metal wear silk gloves which give good protection without interfering with fine sensation of touch. Skin, especially when wet, sticks to metal and may be pulled off when trying to remove your hand. For the same reason never put your tongue against freezing metal.

d. Feet. Tight boots cramp the circulation of blood and cause blisters. Once the surface of normal skin is broken the tissues are more liable both to cold injury and infection. Tie laces loosely because if they freeze and are difficult to undo you may not bother to stop and remove your boots as soon as your feet begin to feel cold or to lose sensation. Warming them early may prevent serious trouble later. Wet socks quickly lose their warmth so always carry a spare dry pair. Wear gaiters to keep snow out of your boots and keep your feet dry. A sock will wrinkle if it sinks down into a boot making uneven 'pressure areas' where blood supply is reduced, making the foot liable to frostbite.

How?

To understand the mechanism of frostbite a knowledge of the structure and function of blood vessels is helpful. Blood pumped from the heart passes through tubes of ever-decreasing calibre — aorta, arteries and arterioles — until it reaches the skin capillaries.

Arterioles, the smaller arteries on the out-going side of the circulation, have smooth muscle in their walls under reflex nervous control. In response to stimulation by heat they become larger in calibre (vaso-dilatation) or in cold they clamp down (vaso-constriction). Small bands of smooth muscle wrapped round the junction of the arteriole and capillary tighten in response to cold and allow blood to by-pass the capillary circulation. This blood is shunted direct from arteriole to venule and does not lose heat at the cold skin surface. This is one of Nature's ways of keeping the vital core temperature of the body normal; the odd limb is expendable and can be sacrificed to frostbite at your inconvenience, but if the body core temperature falls too low you die.

Capillaries are minute vessels with walls one single cell thick and no muscle fibres in them. They are not under the control of the nervous system. Blood flow in the capillaries is regulated, like lock-gates, by the amount of blood released into them by the arterioles and is manifest in the colour of the skin, which varies from healthy pink to ashen pallor. The capillary bed can hold a large volume

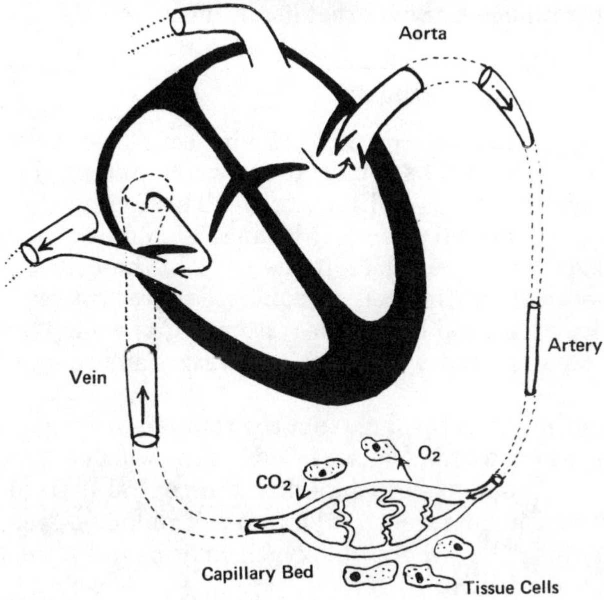

Figure 17.1 Blood circulation

of blood which flows just under the skin so heat is readily lost by convection to the outside air. Cold reduces the calibre of the capillaries by causing their lining cells to swell.

Blood empties from the capillaries into venules and then into the larger veins through which it is returned to the heart by means of the negative suction pressure that develops in the chest when you breathe, a system of one-way valves in the veins and the pumping action of the leg muscles.

All the tissues of the body, whether skin, muscle or blood vessels, are built up of cells the function of which is controlled by a nucleus that depends on oxygen for life. Nine-tenths of any cell consists of water in which many chemicals and enzymes are dissolved, and the cells are surrounded by water that lies in the supporting framework.

Mechanism of Frostbite

Below $-1°C$ fluid surrounding the cells freezes slowly forming ice crystals which draw water out of the cell through the intact cell membrane. This upsets the delicate physical and chemical balance of the cell which is damaged or even killed. If ice outside the cells can be thawed before the cell is damaged water moves back into it and normal balance is restored. If the temperature falls rapidly, fluid within the cell freezes and the nucleus dies.

Cold blood returning from the temperature-regulating centres in the brain causes intense narrowing of the arterioles in order to keep blood in the central core of the body and maintain its temperature. If blood vessels constrict thus, the supply of oxygen may be insufficient to keep the cell alive.

Act.

A frostbitten climber may also be suffering from exposure and fatigue. Make him warm, comfortable and free from pain and anxiety before beginning to treat the isolated part of the body that is frozen.

Frostbite, like skin burns, may be superficial or deep according to the layer of cells that is damaged. The depth of freezing depends on the temperature and the length of exposure to cold.

i. Superficial — Frozen white, but soft on pressure. Superficial freezing ('frostnip' or 'frostnumb' (Rosedale)) damages only the surface cells and complete healing with no loss of tissue can be expected. The frozen area is white or waxy and feels intensely cold with tingling pain and numbness. The flesh is soft and resilient when pressed on. Pain indicates that the nerves have *not* been damaged and that the injury is superficial.

Frostnumb is the only form of frostbite that should, and must, be treated out on the mountain. Exercise to get warm. Wriggle toes, flex ankles or place a foot against the warm body of a fit (and, you hope, understanding) companion. Clap hands together, swing arms or put a hand in your own armpit or crutch. If ears or nose feel numb ask a friend to spare some of his hot breath to warm them. Avoid rubbing the skin vigorously because of the danger of breaking the surface and introducing infection. Never rub snow onto the frozen part because the crystals are sharp and abrade the skin.

Numbness wears off as you thaw out, so pain-killing drugs will be necessary to relieve the intense feeling of burning.

ii. Deep — Frozen white, blue or black tissue; solid on pressure. Deep frostbite kills tissue. Damage ranges from a patch of black skin to gangrene and loss of a whole limb; it starts insidiously with loss of pain and cold sensation, indicating that nerves have been injured. Other deep structures such as muscle will also be affected, but tendons are usually spared as is shown by the fact that frostbitten limbs are still capable of movement. The ugly appearance of frostbite is a poor guide to the amount of tissue that will die ultimately. At first the skin is a mottled blue colour and blisters form under the surface. If the limb can be kept absolutely immobile do not risk infection by pricking or lancing blisters which will dry up of their own accord over several weeks and form a black crusted scab. Cover the wound with a plain dry non-stick dressing. If he has to use the limb and will therefore break the blisters anyway, lance, de-roof and dress them meticulously.

A frozen limb swells and becomes tight so it is difficult to move. Raise it on a bundle of clothes or a rucksack above the level of the body in order to let the oedema fluid drain away. If you are patient and do no more than rest the limb and keep it clean, dead slough will separate from healthy healing tissue. The cells on the edge of an area of frostbite are in a precarious balance between life and death; you must try to ensure they survive and keep further damage to a minimum.

Try to keep a frostbitten climber walking on frozen feet under his own power since, once frozen, the feet will suffer no progressive damage. If the limb thaws and then freezes again the cells are further damaged and more tissue dies. Keep a thawed limb warm, at rest, and protected from injury. In this state a climber becomes a cripple and cannot help himself off the mountain. He will probably have to be carried on a stretcher or evacuated by helicopter and the retreat of the entire party will be slowed, with all the dangers this entails. In remote regions where evacuation may take several days the frostbitten climber will have to rest at night. Rewarming is then inevitable so you will just have to manage as best you can.

When the casualty reaches base camp or shelter with adequate after-care facilities, rewarm him thoroughly (see page 45) before attempting to thaw his frozen limb. Keep the room very warm, dress him in dry clothes and place him in a sleeping bag with hot-water-bottles or stones heated in the fire, well-wrapped in clothing to avoid contact burns. Give him plenty of hot drinks. A nip of whisky or brandy with some glucose sweets or drink (see page 45) will cheer him and raise his morale; he will have to be blind drunk on strong alcohol before he loses a significant amount of heat owing to blood vessels dilating. But forbid cigarettes because nicotine severely constricts blood vessels; one puff of a fag can reduce the calibre of small and middle-sized arteries by half.

Act.

i. Rapid thawing. Much of the damage caused by frostbite occurs during thawing. Ice formed between the cells turns into water and chemicals move across the walls upsetting the cell's function.

Rapid but cautious thawing has been shown to be the best treatment for frostbite. Less tissue is damaged than by slow rewarming; blood starts to circulate again after a period of stagnation and carries away the chemical solutions formed during thawing; the freezing time is reduced and swelling, which is inevitable during thawing, subsides more quickly.

Rapid thawing can only be done at a base camp where adequate fuel and large containers are available for heating sufficient water. Immerse the limb in water at 40–44°C for 20 minutes; if the temperature rises above 44°C more tissue will be damaged. A cold limb cools the water so the temperature must be kept up by gradually adding more warm water and stirring. If you do not have a low-reading thermometer (which should be carried in every expedition medical kit), a useful guide is that the water should feel pleasantly warm to the uninjured hand and forearm which are generously provided with heat-sensitive nerves.

Never thaw a frozen limb in front of an open flame as you will just cook the flesh. If warm water is not available thaw the limb by placing it against the body of a healthy, carefully chosen, companion — this is a good test of friendship.

ii. Pain-killing drugs. Give full doses of morphine before thawing. Beware if the victim has a head injury, chest injury, is suffering from exposure or has difficulty with breathing from any other cause, because this drug depresses breathing.

iii. Vaso-dilator drugs ('Ronicol', 'Priscol'). These have *no* place in the treatment of frostbite. The vessels dilate under their influence giving a deceptively pleasant feeling of warmth as a rush of blood surges to the skin surface; but much heat is thereby lost from the central body core with the consequent danger of hypothermia.

Take meticulous care to avoid infection after thawing. A dry scab with a clear line of demarcation between healthy and dead tissue will separate by itself in due course; infection will convert it into a soggy inflamed gangrene that spreads up the limb destroying as it goes. The black scab that is so tempting to pick at protects healing tissue underneath.

After thoroughly washing your own hands with soap and boiled water, clean the frostbitten area with a dilute antiseptic solution. Gentle dabbing is sufficient; do not hurt the skin surface by scrubbing. If the line of demarcation becomes inflamed and tender with spreading redness and throbbing give one of the broad spectrum antibiotics, ampicillin, tetracycline or co-trimoxazole.

All your efforts must be directed towards getting the casualty to hospital where he can receive specialist care. Amputation may then be necessary, only as a last resort, for the control of infection. Eschew heroic surgery in the field; you can only guess at the extent of irreparable damage and notoriously evil-looking limbs can, and do, recover completely.

SNOWBLINDNESS

Snowblindness is caused by an ultra-violet burn of the cornea. Sunlight reflects strongly off snow and light-coloured rocks; its rays can penetrate hazy cloud and

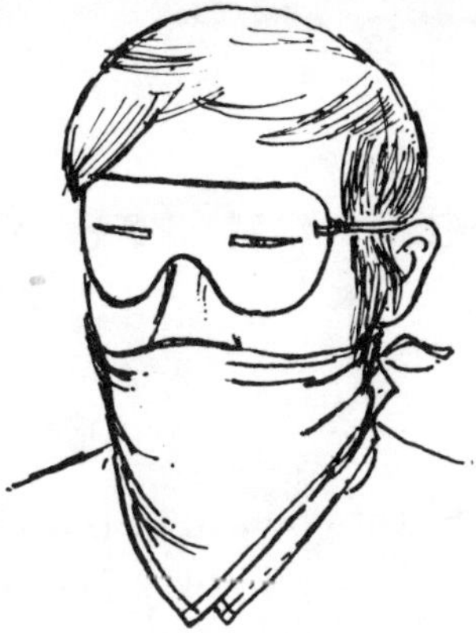

Figure 17.2 Home-made goggles and silk scarf

they become more powerful the higher you climb. The result is intense pain so the eyes are screwed up tightly, and such swelling of the conjunctiva and blistering of the cornea that the victim cannot see out. He becomes temporarily 'blind' and has to be led or carried to a lower camp on the mountain, which may endanger the lives of his companions. Snowblindness can be prevented by wearing goggles or dark glasses with side-shields to exclude glare. In an emergency horizontal slits cut in a piece of cardboard and tied round the head by a piece of string (after the standard Eskimo pattern of snow goggle) allows full protection and ample vision. A silk scarf over the lower face prevents sunburn.

Act.

Anaesthetic drops may relieve the pain and spasm for long enough to let the casualty reach camp unaided. Thereafter both eyes are treated as severe corneal abrasions and the victim becomes a stretcher case.

18

Foreign Travel

Immunization

When travelling abroad you can be protected by immunization against certain infectious diseases common in tropical and sub-tropical countries. Inoculation with a small amount of the organism or a purified derivative of the toxin that causes the disease, though not enough to give you the disease, stimulates your body to produce immune antibodies that mop up stray and dangerous bugs.

Protection against typhoid, paratyphoid and tetanus is an advisable safeguard wherever you go abroad, and inoculations can be done by your family doctor. Immunization against poliomyelitis, diphtheria and tuberculosis is given to most schoolchildren and need not be repeated, but you should check that this was done in childhood.

Immunization against smallpox, yellow fever and cholera is at present compulsory by international agreement, and you have to show a valid up-to-date International Certificate at the place of entry to many countries abroad, and this can apply to short stop-overs while in transit during the main journey. The certificate has to be on an approved form, signed and dated by the doctor who inoculated you, and stamped by the local authority of your area. You will also have to produce valid International Certificates when returning to the United Kingdom from most countries abroad. The embassy of the country concerned will give you the most recent information on inoculation requirements.

If in doubt about any aspects of immunization enquire at your District Community Physician's Department (Public Health Department).

A. Compulsory Inoculations (International Certificate required)

i. Smallpox. The disease is endemic in India, East Africa and parts of the Far East, but occurs sporadically throughout the world. Vaccination, by lightly scratching the skin with a sharp needle, can be done by your family doctor, but the certificate he will give you must be stamped by the local authority. After the first (primary) vaccination a blister develops in 3–4 days and may take several weeks to heal, leaving a small permanent scar which proves that vaccination has 'taken'. Revaccination makes less mark, has to be done every three years, and the certificate must be properly signed and stamped each time.

Because of the danger of adverse reactions to vaccination, people who suffer from eczema or violent allergy, pregnant women, and those taking steroid medicines are exempt, but need a medical certificate from their doctor.

ii. Yellow fever used to be a common killing disease in the forests of Central and South America, and East, Central and West Africa, but it is now quite rare. Mosquitos carry the disease from mammals, principally monkeys, to man.

Immunization is compulsory for people travelling to or through an endemic area. Inoculation by one single injection must be done at least 5 days before Smallpox (preferably 3 weeks), never at the same time, and only in officially designated centres. The certificate is valid 10 days after immunization and lasts 10 years.

iii. Cholera. This serious water-borne bowel infection causes profuse watery diarrhoea, cramps and collapse.

The patient can die in a few hours from loss of water.

Immunization will soon no longer need an International Certificate as it only gives partial protection. But certain countries still require evidence of immunization. Care of drinking water and food is more important in prevention. Immunization is given only immediately before visiting, or passing through, an infected area and should be reserved for such an occasion. It is given by two deep subcutaneous injections of 0.5 ml., spaced 4–6 weeks apart and immunity only lasts 6 months.

B. Advisable Inoculations (not compulsory).

i. Tetanus. 'Lockjaw' still occurs in Britain and is not uncommon abroad. Prevention by a course of immunization is simple, but treatment may be very unpleasant.

Spores of the organism that causes tetanus lie dormant in the soil, particularly where horse and sheep manure abound. They enter through a break in the skin after even a trivial wound or animal bite and especially when there has been much destruction of tissue. Thorough cleaning of the wound and removal of dead tissue is mandatory.

For active immunization three 0.5 ml. doses of *adsorbed* tetanus toxoid (dried inactivated serum) are given by intramuscular injection, 4–6 weeks elapsing between the first and second injections, and 6–12 months between the second and third. Most children are covered by their 'triple' diphtheria/pertussis/tetanus (DPT) immunization course which is complete by the age of 18 months. All persons who have been immunized should carry a card to say when this was last done so they can be checked in case of an accident with a dirty wound. After a wound an immunized person should have a 'booster' dose of 0.5 ml. of adsorbed toxoid; otherwise a booster is needed every five years to keep up safe immunity.

If a person has not been immunized before (and if he

cannot remember, it is best to regard him as starting again from scratch) a prophylactic injection of 1 ml. of human tetanus immunoglobulin should be given once at the same time as starting a course of tetanus toxoid. There is nowadays no place for the use of anti-tetanus horse serum (ATS) in the routine prevention of tetanus.

The tetanus organism is sensitive to several antibiotics and effective if started soon after the injury. Penicillin and tetracycline are the drugs of choice. Antibiotics are often given routinely for prevention at the same time as tetanus toxoid.

ii. Typhoid and Paratyphoid. These diseases are carried by infected water and food so scrupulous care with drinking water and preparation of food is the best precaution.

Monovalent anti-typhoid serum is used for immunization as it has fewer side-effects than the old T.A.B.T. and protection against paratyphoid A and B is now thought to be ineffective. Two subcutaneous injections are given spaced 7–28 days apart. A third dose 6–12 months later completes the primary course. A reinforcing 'booster' dose is given every year if you go abroad frequently, or every 3 years if you just want to keep your immunity up to date. An intradermal (into the skin) injection uses a smaller dose and causes a less severe reaction. Pain and stiffness in the arm, headache and generally feeling rotten are common side effects. Avoid alcohol for a day or two afterwards. Tetanus toxoid cover can be given at the same time.

iii. Diphtheria, Tuberculosis and Poliomyelitis. Immunization is given to most schoolchildren and lasts a lifetime. You are probably protected, but it is wise to check with your family doctor.

Poliomyelitis virus is passed in the faeces. Insanitary conditions in mountain huts have been the probable cause of several serious cases among mountaineers in recent years. Take a reinforcing dose (on a sugar lump) if you are going to be living rough, especially in the tropics, for a long time.

B.C.G. immunization against TB, which is still common in some underdeveloped countries, is given to people who have a negative reaction to Heaf or Mantoux skin sensitivity testing.

iv. Infectious Hepatitis. This virus infection is usually carried in faeces and acquired from infected food and water, or by swimming near a sewage outlet. Jaundice, a yellow discolouration of the skin most easily noticed in the whites of the eyes, is preceded by a vague and unpleasant malaise for 2–3 weeks, and the person often feels better once the jaundice has appeared.

No preventive immunization exists. Gamma (Immuno-) globulin gives some protection if given within two weeks of exposure to the virus, so should be reserved for recent contacts and not given as long-term protection. It is very expensive.

v. Malaria. Anopheline mosquitos transmit parasites which cause malaria. The symptoms are high fever, shivering, aching and sweats. No immunization is possible against malaria. Although it has been eradicated from many parts of the world there are still large areas of the tropics where malaria is endemic. The Anopheline species carries malaria and tends to bite around dusk. At rest it appears to be standing on its head with its body at an angle to the surface whereas the Culicine (nuisance only) mosquito stands horizontally. Discourage them from biting by wearing long sleeves and trousers, by using insect repellant and sleeping under mosquito netting at night. But you cannot entirely avoid bites and it only takes one bite from an infected mosquito to pass on malaria. So

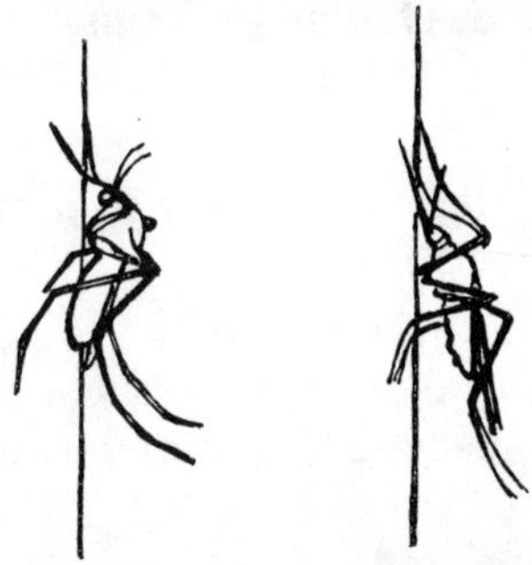

Figure 18.1 Malaria mosquitos

anti-malarial medicines are the only true protection.

Prophylactic anti-malarial drugs suppress malarial parasites introduced into the blood stream provided the concentration of drug is kept high enough by regular use.

The following is a schedule of anti-malarial prevention:

Name	Trade name	Tablet strength	Number	Frequency	Minimum time before departure
Proguanil	('Paludrine')	100 mg	1	daily	1 day
Pyrimethamine	('Daraprim')	25 mg	1	weekly	1 day
Chloroquine	('Nivaquine')	100 mg	3	weekly	1 day

N.B.

— Drugs should be taken with liquid after a meal.

— Start taking anti-malarial drugs one week before arriving in the malarial area, take them throughout the visit, and continue for 4–6 weeks after returning home.

— Although taking a drug weekly is convenient, you are less likely to forget a daily dose if it becomes a habit like cleaning your teeth. One single omission interrupts the protective effect, so forgetting a weekly dose could be serious.

— Even making a brief stop-over in a malarial country you need full protection.

— Ask a doctor on arrival what is the best prophylactic drug for the area in case there is a particularly virulent or resistant local species. You may be advised to double the dose if there is.

If you develop an unexplained fever in the tropics or after return, consult a doctor and ask for a blood film examination. This should be done especially on returning home from a malarious area. (The Ross Institute of Tropical Hygiene, Keppel Street, London WC1E 7HT). Always tell a doctor you may have to consult that you have recently been in the tropics.

PRECAUTIONS AGAINST INFECTIOUS ORGANISMS

Water and food are the most common sources of disease because they become polluted by infected faeces and the urine of a carrier, e.g. typhoid, dysentery, cholera, schistosomiasis, hookworm. Generally speaking people in tropical countries are less discriminating about where they defaecate, partly owing to ignorance, partly to lack of adequate latrines. Germs from an infected person may directly contaminate the drinking water supplies, or are carried to food by flies. These diseases are prevented by drinking only pure water, eating clean food and disposing of sewerage efficiently.

A. Water

Infected drinking water causes many problems. If in doubt about the water, purify it yourself. In most clean hotels and restaurants abroad the water is safe to drink, and often drinking water on the tables has been purified. Water taken direct from the taps is best avoided and certain towns (e.g. Kathmandu) are notorious for polluted civil water supplies.

Hillside springs, well clear of human habitation and animal grazing, should be safe, but stream and river water is likely to be polluted. Glacial mud and mica that give alpine rivers their murky appearance often upset the gut.

Water Purification

1. Boiling. Boiling briskly for a few seconds kills most organisms (including amoeba cysts and infectious hepatitis virus) and is the only way water can be truly 'sterilized'. The colour, taste and smell of water is immaterial provided it has been boiled. (This may be a problem at high altitude where the boiling point is lower than at sea-level so boiling takes longer and is less efficient.) A wise rule is to drink tea or coffee that has been made with boiling water.

2. Chemical treatment. Chlorine is the basic ingredient of most water-purifying tablets which are useful for disinfecting most water-borne bacteria, but will not touch amoeba cysts or bacteria embedded in solid particles. Iodine kills amoeba cysts as well as bacteria.

When large quantities of water have to be prepared and boiling is not practicable purifying tablets, which can be bought from any chemist, can be put in the water bottles, but they leave a taste of chlorine. The directions for use are printed on the bottle.

3. Filtration. Filters (Milipore, Katadyn, Millbank Filter bag) remove suspended matter and some bacteria, giving the water a deceptively clear appearance. They are useful for cleaning large amounts of water but are the least reliable way of making it pure. Filters have to be kept scrupulously clean or they lose their value. Water should be boiled after filtration, not before.

B. Drinks

Bottled fizz, iced drink cubes and ice-lollies are only as safe as the water from which they are made, is clean. Milk must be boiled if not pasteurised; powdered milk is safe if made up with boiled water but should then only be kept in a refrigerator. Wine drunk in moderation is harmless but a surfeit upsets the stomach. Spirits have to be taken in excessive amounts in order to kill any germs; there are more efficient but possibly less pleasant ways of doing this.

C. Ice Cream

Germs are harboured notoriously in ice-cream both from the ingredients and from subsequent handling. Well advertised brands cannot afford to lose their reputation by slackness in their preparation and so should be reasonably safe.

D. Food

Freshly and thoroughly cooked food is safe since any bacteria will have been killed by the heat; so avoid precooked and handled food, especially where flies abound. Peel all fruit and vegetables; thorough washing is only second best so beware of salads, tomatoes, lettuces and especially watercress because human nightsoil is often used as a fertilizer in the tropics. Meat should be thoroughly cooked and eaten immediately as raw or underdone beef and pork harbour tapeworms. Risk shell-fish and inadequately cleaned prawns only if you have a tough stomach.

You have to strike a balance between making life a misery through worrying about what you eat and drink and taking commonsense precautions. You cannot shield your gut from every conceivable germ, and some early contact, with its resulting dose of the 'runs', is inevitable to allow yourself to build up immunity that will protect you from further attacks.

E. Hygiene

Many toilets are dirty; you may have to squat and keep your balance by holding on to the walls. Take your own toilet paper as newsprint is rough and fragile. Wash your hands carefully with soap as soon as possible afterwards. Remember, dirty lavatories = dirty kitchens.

Brush your teeth in boiled water only. Chewing gum is a useful temporary freshener when clean water is scarce.

GUT

Traveller's Diarrhoea

Known at home as 'food poisoning' or 'gastro-enteritis', this illness *causes more trouble to the traveller than all the other medical hazards abroad put together.* It has as many local names (Gippy Tummy, Delhi Belly, Kathmandu Quickstep, Tokyo Trots, Rangoon Runs, Montezuma's Revenge) as patent remedies. The causes are usually untraceable but may include gluttony, change in climate, and an upset in the bacteria that are normal and necessary in the bowel. Frank infection with disease-causing organisms carried in water and food is less common.

Much pleasure in travelling abroad comes from eating local food and drinking wine; it is hardly worth going all that way for beer, fish and chips. But be moderate to avoid what could turn out to be a very expensive tummy upset that will spoil your journey.

Act.

Traveller's diarrhoea is usually a self-limiting illness that clears in 2-3 days. You may vomit and feel groggy because of dehydration due to loss of body water. Go to bed and drink unlimited fluids (at least a pint an hour of plain boiled water). Avoid eating except dried toast, peeled grated apple turned brown (pectin) or kaolin powder. A short period of starvation can do you no harm and the idea that you must 'give the stomach something to work on' is nonsense.

The 'Everest Blunderbuss Cocktail' constipates most people for a week.

Recipe:—	Kaolin powder	2 tablespoons.
	Codeine phosphate 15 mg.	2–4 tablets.
	Diphenoxylate, ('Lomotil')	4–6 tablets.
	Tincture of morphine, ('Chlorodyne')	4–6 drops (sleepy-making)

Antibiotics should not be used blindly since they kill normal bacteria, which are protective, as well as poison-producing ones; they play little part in speeding recovery and may prolong the excretion of bugs during convalescence. Many popular brands of diarrhoea medicine are at best useless, at worst potentially dangerous.

If diarrhoea does not stop on this treatment, or if blood appears in the stools, consult a doctor. If this is impossible because of geographical isolation, the best initial drug is co-trimoxazole or a simple sulphonamide.

Dysentery

Infection of the bowel with bacteria or amoeba can only be diagnosed accurately by examining the stool under the microscope and by growing the offending organism. Antibiotic sensitivity can then be tested and the appropriate drug prescribed.

a. Bacillary dysentery. Salmonella, shigella (which also causes typhoid) and staphylococci are the usual organisms of the disease, which is commoner than amoebic dysentery.

The onset is acute and severe. The temperature rises quickly to 38° - 39°C and the patient feels sick but usually does not vomit. He has urgent, explosive diarrhoea that may contain blood and mucus, and cramps in his abdomen.

Act.

Consult a doctor who may prescribe sulpha drugs or chloramphenicol (many doctors who have not suffered themselves may disapprove of using this drug).

b. Amoebic dysentery. Amoebic dysentery is much rarer and has a more gradual onset than bacillary dysentery and may take more than a month to develop. Each day 3–4 loose foul-smelling stools are passed, increasing to a dozen with blood, a lot of mucus, painful straining and colic.

Act.

Metronidazole is the drug of choice.

Typhoid (Enteric) Fever

Infection is caused by the germ salmonella typhi. Fever increases in a spiky fashion over several weeks, with bloody diarrhoea and headache. Eventually the patient is prostrate and desperately ill.

Act.

Medical help is urgently needed. Chloramphenicol is the drug of choice; prednisone taken for a week reduces the symptoms rapidly and makes the dangerous complication of perforation of the bowel less likely.

Cholera

Cholera was epidemic throughout the world in 1973, notably in parts of Italy. The cholera organisms come only from the human intestine and are spread by faecally contaminated water, not by direct contact or inhalation. Raw shellfish collect the germs and are particularly dangerous.

A sudden onset of profuse watery diarrhoea with cramps and ultimate collapse due to dehydration (which can all happen within a few hours) in a known epidemic area calls for immediate attention at hospital.

Act.

Fluid should be replaced by intravenous drip, whenever possible. The antibiotics of choice are tetracycline and chloramphenicol.

Worms

Most worms can be prevented by careful hygiene and by boiling drinking water. An itchy bottom is often the first warning; look carefully for the worm, or part of it, in your stool. Usually one dose of the appropriate anti-parasitic drug cleans out the worms.

i. Roundworms and Threadworms. These worms are easily seen. They can mimic appendicitis and, as this is rare in natives of the tropics, doctors should beware of wielding the knife unnecessarily.
Drug. Piperazine.

ii. Tapeworms. Tapeworms thrive in under-cooked beef, pork and fish. Segments of the worm are passed in the stool, but the head remains attached to the gut and must be killed to prevent it growing again.
Drug. Dichlorophen.

iii. Hookworms. Larvae enter through abrasions in the feet, so you should wear shoes in an infected area. Blood in the stool and anaemia occur.
Drug. Bephenium granules.

iv. Bilharzia (Schistosomiasis). The fluke lives in fresh water in Africa, Central America and Japan. It enters the body by drinking infected water or through the feet so beware of paddling in or drinking from slow-flowing rivers and lakes. The veins of the bladder are its favourite haunt so passing blood in the urine is a danger sign; diarrhoea and itching are frequent.
Drugs — should be under supervision of a doctor.

Constipation

Constipation is rarely a problem when travelling abroad. Drink plenty, and eat fruit and roughage; if this does not help take a laxative. In desperation give an enema by passing a pint of soapy solution into the rectum using a well-greased rubber tube and a funnel.

SKIN

Fungus Infections

a. Athlete's Foot. Scales and cracks begin in the clefts between the small toes and the skin becomes white and moist. Itching is awful.

Act.

Carefully wash and dry between the toes with a towel kept exclusively for your own use. Powder the feet with an anti-fungal powder but cream may be better in the acute stages of the infection. Use open sandals, but if socks are necessary wear cotton rather than nylon, and change them frequently.

b. Dhobie Itch. The groin is infected by the same fungus, and the area is red, clearly edged and itches badly.

Act.

As above, but read 'groin' for 'feet'.

Bites

i. Animals. After any animal bite, however small, you should have a tetanus toxoid booster. In the tropics rabies must always be considered.

Rabies. Though dogs are the commonest vectors, foxes, wolves, cats, bats, and various other animals can carry the rabies virus. The virus only enters humans through a break in the skin. It lives in the saliva of an infected animal whose nervous system becomes affected, causing the 'frothing of mad dogs'.

If bitten or licked by a suspect animal wash the wound with copious soap and water, but not so vigorously as to break the skin. If the wound is left open to the sun, ultra-violet light may kill any virus remaining after washing.

A course of anti-rabies vaccine with 20 daily injections into the skin of the abdomen lasts 2 weeks, so will not be undertaken lightly. The suspected animal should, if possible, be caged to see if it develops signs of rabies. If it is alive 10 days after the suspicious bite the patient cannot have rabies. If the animal shows signs of illness let it die or kill it and have the brain examined by a laboratory for rabies virus within 24 hours.

There is no known treatment for rabies, and once truly diagnosed, no hope of recovery.

ii. Snakes. If snakes are known to be in the area wear boots, examine them and your sleeping bag before climbing in, and use a torch in the dark. Snakes only attack people when frightened or provoked. Only bites from poisonous snakes cause dangerous snake-bite poisoning, and only one out of 10 people bitten by poisonous snakes die.

If someone is bitten take him to the local hospital which will probably keep anti-venom against the local varieties of poisonous snake. Kill the snake for accurate identification if you can. In the meantime try to reduce the amount of venom entering the circulating blood.

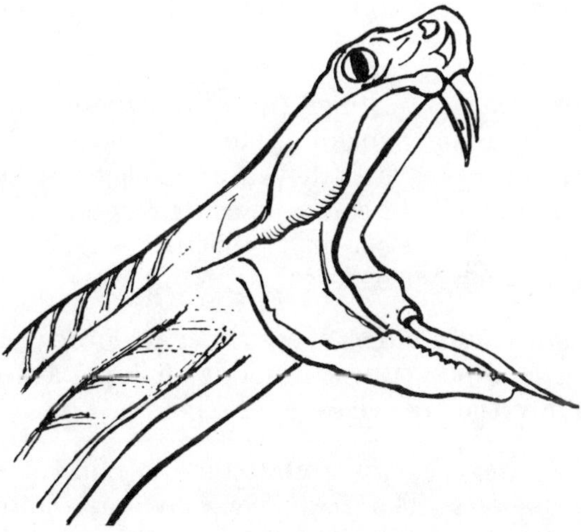

Figure 18.2 Viper with 2 fangs

Wash the bite thoroughly with soap and water. If a hospital is more than an hour away or if the limb starts to swell, immediately tie a handkerchief or other constricting bandage above and below the bite to close off veins and lymph vessels that return blood, and hence poison, to the heart. The 'tourniquet' must not be tight enough to occlude arteries and it must be released every half hour. The toes and fingers should remain pink and warm. Do not cut the skin over the bite or urinate on it as the old wives' tale tells.

Carry the victim so that his circulation is not speeded by exercise; splint the bitten limb and keep it dependent to localize the poison.

Anti-venom is horse serum that neutralizes the injected poison; it can cause severe reactions so must be reserved for potentially serious bites.

If cobra venom has been spat in the eyes, wash them out with copious water.

Pain must be treated and reassurance given as snake bites strike terror into the heart of the most courageous person.

iii. Wasps and Bees. Stings from both these can be extremely painful and shocking. The part swells and itches. The stings of wasps are relieved by vinegar, of bees (B) by bicarbonate (B) of soda. An acute reaction (anaphylaxis) can follow a sting in a sensitive person; this is a medical emergency (see later page 192).

iv. Scorpions and Spiders. These bites are more venomous than wasp or bee stings. Emetine or local anaesthetic injected into the area gives rapid relief.

v. Leeches. Leeches are troublesome in rain forests and tropical marshes. The first sign may be a bootful of blood at the end of the day since the bite is painless and contains a substance that prevents clotting. Leeches find their way into the most carefully laced boots, so open sandals may be an advantage so they can be seen early. Salt or a lighted cigarette makes the leech drop off; do not pull them off or the head will be left in the wound.

vi. Black fly. Black fly are so tiny they penetrate mosquito netting, and give a vicious bite out of proportion to their size. They are world-wide but particularly troublesome in subarctic regions. No protection is of avail.

vii. Fleas. Fleas cause intense itching and a trail of bites usually left around the midriff. They have brown bodies flattened from front to the back, which is bristled.

viii. Lice. Lice are small grey creatures that live in hair and clothing. If you search hard the eggs can be seen attached to the roots of hairs on the head or in the pubic area.

ix. Bedbugs. Bedbugs bite and smell, though they do not carry disease.

x. Scabies. The mites that cause scabies tunnel between the fingers and at other creases. They are often recognized by the scratch marks caused by the intense itching and tiny red spots at the point of entry. Benzyl benzoate kills the mites in the skin.

Insects

Insecticides. Crystals of powder or droplets of spray stick to the insect and slowly paralyse it. The clothing and the person must be treated. The best insecticides contain:-

DDT (Dicophane)
HCH. ('Gammexane')

Insect repellents. These are applied to the skin and are effective for a maximum of four hours, after which they need to be reapplied. The best repellents contain:-

DET (Diethyl toluamide) 'Flypel', 'Skeet-o-stick'.
DMP (Dimethyl phthalate) 'Dimp'.
DBP (Dibutyl phthalate).

Anti-itch. Itching can almost literally drive you crazy; the more you scratch the more you itch. Scratching with dirty finger nails is likely to turn a bite septic.

a. Calamine lotion is more soothing and cooling than the cream, but is more bulky to carry.

b. Anti-histamines all have a powerful anti-itch effect but are also soporific; chlorpheniramine less than most. Beware of anti-histamine creams as they sensitize the skin to anti-histamine medicines taken later, and a violent skin reaction may result.

c. Steroid cream is also effective against itching if other methods fail.

Allergy. Severe allergic (anaphylactic) reactions may follow bites, stings or injections to which the person is sensitive. The patient may begin with the mild symptoms of the bite but rapidly become shocked with severe tightness in the chest and wheezing, and abdominal pain that makes him vomit.

Act.

Hydrocortisone should be injected, if possible, into a vein and the patient treated for shock (q.v.). Adrenaline is a good drug in competent hands but it has dangerous effects on the heart if not carefully administered.

SUN

a. Sunburn. The sun can be a stealthy enemy; if reflects strongly off water, sand and snow, and burning rays can penetrate hazy cloud and are more powerful the higher the altitude. Those with fair skin, red hair or freckles are prone to sunburn, but people vary in the speed with which they tan; tanned skin is the best skin protection. Ideally allow yourself less than an hour in the sun the first day and increase the time gradually. Falling asleep in the sun is a sure way to fry yourself and even a solar-topee won't save mad dogs or Englishmen.

Sun creams and lotions act as a screen to bar the ultraviolet rays from the skin; none of them speed 'le bronzage'. They may reduce burning (and tanning at the same time) but with excessive sun they merely act as fat in the process of frying. Rationing sunlight on your skin, especially unaccustomed areas, is cheaper and more effective. A wide-brimmed hat and a beard give good protection, but lips and noses burn easily and need cover, especially on the underside, from ultraviolet light reflected off snow.

Several 'ultraviolet barrier', 'sunscreens', and 'glacier creams' are available.

Para-aminobenzoic esters ('Spectraban', 'Soltan').

Mexenone ('Uvistat').

'Sylvasun' tablets contain Vitamin A which antagonizes Vitamin D and encourages excessive formation of Vitamin D which protects the skin from burning sunlight, without reducing tanning.

Act.

If the skin goes shrimp-pink and feels prickly and hot, stay in the shade or wear a hat or loose clothing when it is necessary to go out in the sun. Calamine is soothing;

lotion has a cooling effect but is not as convenient as cream. Antihistamines allay itching but may be soporific; antihistamine creams should not be used because of sensitivity reactions. If the skin turns bright lobster and blisters it is badly burnt and a cream containing a steroid is useful.

Treat blisters in the usual way but make sure they remain clean. If a severe general body upset with headache, vomiting and fainting develops due to sunburn, the patient should go to bed and keep cool.

b. Prickly heat. An uncomfortable, itching heat rash develops in sweaty places where air is excluded (armpits, elbow angles, groins, backs of knees) or where clothing is tight or rubs the skin.

Act.

Wear loose clothing and light bed cover at night. Shower frequently using soap, and dry carefully. A dusting powder (boric acid, zinc oxide) or calamine lotion relieves itching. Alcohol encourages skin vessels to dilate and makes itching worse.

c. Heat cramp and heat exhaustion. This usually follows heavy and prolonged exercise in unacclimatized new arrivals to sudden heat and is caused by not taking sufficient water and salt to balance losses in sweating. Tiredness, cramps and vomiting are warning signs of impending collapse. The skin becomes dry and inelastic, the tongue is like sandpaper and the urine scanty, cloudy and a deep yellow-brown colour, indicating dehydration.

Act.

Drink large amounts of fluid and take salt as taste dictates when in the tropics. Food seems tasteless until enough salt has been added; concentrated salt tablets should be unnecessary. Avoid alcohol.

If someone has collapsed and cannot drink, fluid can be given by enema in large volumes with absolute safety as the body will only absorb the amount it requires (see p. 104).

Cool the victim slowly over about one hour, as too sudden cooling can be dangerous, and if possible monitor his rectal temperature throughout. Icepacks, tepid sponging, fanning and wrapping in a wet sheet are all methods of cooling. Aspirin lowers the temperature.

If the person has recently returned from a malarious area remember the possibility that his high temperature may be due to malignant tertian malaria.

d. Sunstroke/heatstroke. When the body gets too hot its heat-regulating mechanism packs up, sweating ceases and the temperature rises far above normal because the casualty cannot lose heat fast enough. He becomes acutely short of water and feels thirsty, dizzy and sick; the skin feels hot and dry. Without treatment, the casualty's temperature may rise above (106°F) (41°C) and he becomes confused and may have convulsions; above (110°F) (43°C) he is likely to slip into coma and die. This serious illness warrants urgent medical help.

Act.

Cool the patient rapidly (see above).

MEDICAL PRELIMINARIES

Before embarking on an expedition ("when a party becomes labelled an expedition it means there are a lot too many people" — Tilman) you are wise to have a thorough medical check-up and certain tests, not only to see that you are fit, but also to have a baseline for comparison should you fall ill later. You do not have to be tough and hairy to go on an expedition or be a good outdoorsman, some of the greatest explorers were written off as weaklings in their youth. So beware of excluding good men because of doubtful medical histories that may be no longer relevant.

The examination should include:

a. Past medical history. Serious illnesses, operations (particularly appendicectomy) and drug sensitivity or contact allergies.

Personal medical details can be imprinted on a bracelet or medallion that must be worn constantly (Medic-alert. 43a Wigmore Street London W1H 9LE). This is safer than a card carried in the pocket or wallet, and may be life-saving in an emergency.

e.g. Blood Group — in case blood transfusion is needed after an accident.

Drug treatment dosage — for diabetics, epileptics and those taking steroids or other powerful drugs.

Sensitivity to specific drugs — penicillin, sulphonamides, aspirin.

Allergies — to bites, stings and pollens.

Rare diseases — haemophilia, fragile bones etc.

b. General physical examination and include the following tests;

Urine analysis

Haemoglobin and Blood group

Chest X-ray

c. Dental check.

Remember to take with you;

— Medicines with which you are already being treated. The dosage and pharmacological name should be written on the bottle since proprietary names vary in different countries

— Spare spectacles and your lens prescription.

— Whistle (for girls) in case bottom-pinching gets out of hand. In many countries long hair = hippie, and undeserved rough handling may be given by the police; long hair is also difficult to keep clean. In some places cheap drugs are sold which may be impure and dangerous; the penalties for trafficking are just as severe as at home. VD is commonly associated with drug abuse and alcohol and is rarely caught off cracked cups or lavatory seats. Sometimes the nicest people carry the disease and few of the girls know it. 'Groupies' who walk out to provide creature comforts that may be lacking to expedition members have introduced a new hazard to mountaineering. Any man who has put himself at risk, has a discharge from the penis and passes water painfully and often, should go for a check-up and warn his girlfriend to do likewise.

Oddments that might be useful on an expedition abroad:

Tin trunk
Kit bag, canvas

Poncho groundsheet
Umbrella

Sleeping bag liner
Mattress, closed cell foam
Reindeer/bear skin

Plastic bags, assorted
Zinc oxide plaster tape

Flip-flop sandals/gym shoes
Sun hat
Sun-glasses/goggles

Soap box, plastic
Face wipes

Address cards
Family photograph
Picture book, 'Beautiful Britain'

Pocket note-book
Duplicate books for letters

Urinal, plastic with cap	Clip-board
Nylon line/oiled string	
Machete/axe	Butterfly-net/chemicals
	Flower pressing gear
Egg box, plastic	Dice
Thermos	Playing cards
Hot water bottle	Chess, pocket
Food bags, cotton	Presents:
Pressure cooker	Seeds, (flowers and vegetables)
	Needles, strong
Lemonade powder	Pens, ball-point
Boiled sweets	Balloons

19

Medical Supplies

The medical supplies you carry will be decided by the size of the party, the type of country and your ability to use them; a doctor on a Himalayan expedition and a schoolmaster on the Brecon Beacons have very different needs. Whatever your choice try to spread your medical equipment among several members of the party as the kit is invariably on the other side of the hill at the time it is most urgently needed.

The following scheme is merely a suggestion, but it has several times been proved to work well on the highest mountain in the world.

Each climber has his own small 'individual' medical kit, packed in a waterproof box that lives in the bottom of his rucksack – again, not on the shelf at home. The leader of a small party carries a larger box with more specialized equipment.

On an expedition where the party may be dispersed over the mountain and in neighbouring valleys a 'camp box' should stay in the tents as soon as they are put up, and this box should never be taken from the camp. For forays away from camp take a similar box to tide the party over until their return to camp.

If there is a doctor in the party he will carry his own comprehensive bag and a resuscitation kit as well. The contents will be entirely decided by the personal preference of the doctor and his degree of experience. If you have never done a tracheostomy or given an anaesthetic before it is probably wiser not to start learning in a two-man tent, 20,000 ft. up, in a blizzard. A doctor in the mountains is of use only in proportion to what he knows and understands about the medical problems of mountains, which are highly specialized in their own particular way. Because he has MB, or whatever, after his name it does not mean he is any more use than a competent hillman who has bothered to learn the elements of the trade as it concerns the casualty on the mountainside.

DRUGS AND DRESSINGS

The following list includes only drugs and dressings that have been mentioned in the text of this book. You will have to make up your own list according to your needs, but you should not have to go far beyond the number of items included here. The thinking that has gone behind this choice is summarized thus:

—*Drugs.* All are standard preparations that appear in the British National Formulary (BNF) and are regularly prescribed by doctors. The trade name of proprietary preparations is given when it seems helpful. These are often convenient mixtures of drugs and usually more expensive and no more effective than BNF drugs but sometimes better known to the public. Do not be misled by a well known trade name that slips easily off the tongue (that is what advertising men are paid for) — it may be no better than a common-or-garden household medicine that sounds less exotic e.g. aspirin, penicillin.

— *Simplicity.* If one drug or dressing will do two jobs equally well it avoids reduplication. The less choice you have the easier it may be to decide what to use. Sound hospital medicine is practiced in a very different situation to that faced by a climber on the hill, so you may have to do things that would be frowned on by the pundits.

—*Price.* Being reared by the Welfare State few of us have any idea of the cost of drugs and dressings.

e.g. One 3″ crepe bandage costs (1975) — 0.45p
One 5-day course of 'Septrin' (1975) — £$1.71\frac{1}{2}$p

so 'cheap' medical kits, if they are to be of any use, do not exist.

— *Convenience.* Few liquids are suggested because they are heavy, and bottles break. Small plastic bottles with screw caps are good if a liquid has to be used. The majority of drugs can be taken by mouth. However, if the patient is vomiting, or if there is particular urgency to give a drug, an injection may be necessary, e.g. morphia. Any layman can be taught how to give an injection by a competent nurse better than most doctors, using an orange as a model as it is so like a buttock in form and consistency.

— *Packaging and weight.* If the kit is too heavy you will try very hard to forget it; so keep it light and compact. Strong plastic boxes with water-tight lids can be bought in many shapes and sizes. Pills can be carried in self-sealing plastic envelopes that are easy to write on to label the drugs they hold. Also they take up less space as they become empty.

— *Oxygen.* Oxygen will probably only be carried by ambulances, helicopters, occasional mountain rescue teams and as part of the equipment of high altitude expeditions. It is, however, put in the text where applicable. The same rule applies to 'Entonox'.

PHARMACOPOEIA

Column 1. *Drug group.* For ease of reference these drugs used in a particular medical problem have been grouped together e.g. pain-killers, antibiotics, gut drugs.

Column 2. *Drug name.* The official British National Formulary name is used. This will be understood in most countries of the world. Drugs obtainable only on a doctor's prescription are marked (P); those under the regulations of the Dangerous Drugs Act are marked (DDA).

Column 3. *Proprietary trade name.*

Column 4. *Unit route.* The drug unit is presented as tablet, capsule, injection, suppository etc.

Column 5. *Unit strength.* Each tablet or injection is made up in a certain strength. Where there are alternative strengths the most convenient for the purpose of this book is chosen.

Column 6. *Unit dose.* This shows the number of whatever unit is prescribed that should be taken by a fit adult. *Children's doses are usually half the adult dose*, but vary with the weight of the child.

Column 7. *Daily requirements.* The maximum number of times a day the drug should be taken is shown, and this is the upper limit of the safe dose. Some drugs e.g. antibiotics must be taken for a full course of five days with no short cuts just because the patient appears to be improving.

Column 8. *Cost.* To give a rough guide when choosing your medical kit the cost is given as H (high), M (medium), or L (low).

Side-effects. Most drugs have more or less unpleasant or undesirable side-effects. But in the mountain situation if the drug is needed it must be taken regardless except for the most important side-effects.

1. Group	2. Name (BNF)	3. Trade-Name	4. Unit Route	5. Unit Strength	6. Unit Dose	7. Daily Unit (max.)	8. Cost
Analgesics (pain-killers)							
Mild	Aspirin		tablets	300 mg	1-3	4	L
	– with Codeine	Codis	tablets		1-3	4	L
	Paracetamol	Panadol	tablets	500 mg	1-2	4	L
Moderate	Pentazocine (P)	Fortral	tablets	25 mg	1-4	6	H
			injection	30 mg	1-2	4	H
Strong	Morphine (DDA)		injection	15 mg	1	4	L
Antibiotics (for infection)							
General	Penicillin V (P)		tablets	250 mg	1	4	L
	Sulphadimidine (P)		tablets	500 mg	2	6	L
Broad spectrum	Ampicillin (P)	Penbritin	capsules	250 mg	1-2	4	M
	Co-trimoxazole (P)	Bactrim, Septrin	tablets		1	4	H
	Tetracycline (P)		tablets	250 mg	1	4	L
	Chloramphenicol (P)	Chloromycetin	capsules	250 mg	1	4	M

1. Group	2. Name (BNF)	3. Trade-Name	4. Unit Route	5. Unit Strength	6. Unit Dose	7. Daily Unit (max.)	8. Cost
Anti-amoebic	Metronidazole (P)	Flagyl	tablets	200 mg	2-4	4	H
Sedative (for nerves)							
	Diazepam (P)	Valium	tablets	5 mg	1-2	4	M
(for sleep)						night	
Antihistamines (for itching, allergy, travel sickness)							
	Chlorpheniramine (P)	Piriton	tablets	4 mg	1	4	L
	Promethazine (P)	Phenergan	tablets	25 mg	1	4	L
Lung Relaxants (for wheezing)							
	Aminophylline (P)		suppository	360 mg	1	4	L
	Salbutamol (P)	Ventolin	tablets	4 mg	1-2	4	H
Diuretics (to encourage urine flow)							
	Acetazolamide (P)	Diamox	tablets	250 mg	1	4	H

	Frusemide (P)	Lasix	tablets	40 mg	1	4	H
Steroids (for severe allergy)							
	Prednisone (P)		tablets	5 mg	1-5	4	M
	Hydrocortisone (P)		injection	100 mg	1-3	4	H
Antacids (for indigestion)							
	Aluminium hydroxide		tablets		1-2	4	L
	Magnesium trisilicate		tablets		1-2	4	L
Laxative (for constipation)							
	Senna	Senokot	tablets	7 mg	2-4	1	L
	Bisacodyl	Ducolax	tablets	5 mg	1-2	(night)	M
			suppository		1	(night)	
Anti-Diarrhoea							
	Kaolin		powder	1 tablespoon		4	L
	Codeine phosphate (P)		tablets	15 mg	1	4	L
	Chloroform and morphine	Chlorodyne	tincture	drops	4-6	2	L
	Diphenoxylate (P)	Lomotil	tablets		2-4	4	H

1. Group	2. Name (BNF)	3. Trade-Name	4. Unit Route	5. Unit Strength	6. Unit Dose	7. Daily Unit	8. Cost
Piles							
	Bismuth subgallate	Anusol	suppository		1	2	M
Water Sterilizing							
		Sterotabs Halozone					
Worms							
Roundworms	Piperazine	Antepar	sachet	4 G.	1	1 (after supper)	M
Hookworms	Bephenium	Alcopar	sachet	5 G.	1	1	M
Tapeworm	Dichlorophen	Anthiphen	tablets	500 mg	18	1 (before breakfast)	M
Antimalarial							
	Proguanil	Paludrine	tablets	100 mg	1	1	L
	Pyrimethamine	Daraprim	tablets	25 mg	1	(weekly)	L
	Chloroquine	Nivaquine	tablets	100 mg	3	(weekly)	L

Eyes							
Anaesthetic	Amethocaine (P)		drops	0.25%	1-2	4+	M
Pupil dilator	Homatropine (P)		drops	2.0%	1-2	2	M
Antibiotic	Chloramphenicol (P)	Chloromycetin	drops	0.5%	1-2	4	M
			ointment	1.0%		2	M
Stain	Fluorescein		paper strips				L
Ears							
Antibiotic	Chloramphenicol (P)	Chloromycetin	drops	0.5%	1-2	4	M
Nose							
Decongestant	Ephedrine		drops	1.0%	1-2	4	L
Throat							
Soreness	Benzalkonium		lozenges		1	10	L
	Benzocaine Co.	Tyrozets	lozenges		1	10	L
Teeth							
Dressing	Oil of Cloves		drops			4	M
	Zinc Oxide		powder				L
		Tresiolan					H
		Cavit					H

1. Group	2. Name (BNF)	3. Trade-Name	4. Unit Route	5. Unit Strength	6. Unit Dose	7. Daily Unit (max.)	8. Cost
Crystals (make solution with water)							
Mouth ulcers	Gentian Violet		paint				L
Antiseptic	Potassium Permanganate		paint				L
Exotic	Mercurochrome		paint				L
colours	Brilliant Green		paint				L
	Methylene Blue		paint				L
Antiseptic							
Cleansing	Chlorhexidine		cream				L
	Cetrimide	Savlon	cream				
Drawing pus	Glycerine magnesium sulphate	GMS	paste				L
Soothing	Calamine		lotion cream				L
Steroid							
	Betamethasone (P)	Betnovate	ointment				M
	Fluocinolone (P)	Synalar	ointment				H

Sunscreen				
	Mexenone	Uvistat	cream	H
Rub (For aching muscles)				
	Methyl salicylate and Iodex		ointment	L
Anti-scabies				
	Benzyl benzoate		application	L
Anti-fungus (for athletes foot, dhobie itch)				
	Benzoic acid	Whitfields	ointment	L
	Zinc undecenoate	Tineafax Mycota	cream	L
Insecticide				
	DDT	DDT		L
Insect Repellent				
	Dimethyl-phthalate	Dimp		L

1. Group	2. Name (BNF)	3. Trade-Name	4. Unit Route	5. Unit Strength	6. Unit Dose	7. Daily Unit (max.)	8. Cost
Dressings							
	Plaster dressing strip			36″			L
	Elastoplast			3″ × 5 m			M
	Zinc Oxide plaster			1″ × 5 m			L
		Steristrips		½″ × 4			H
		Dumbells					H
		Anchor Dressings					M
	Bandage Crepe			3″			H
	Cotton			2″			L
	Woven	Krinx or Kling		3″			H
	Gauze Squares			3″ × 3″			
	(plain)						
	(non-stick)	Melolin		4″ × 4″			
	Paraffin Gauze			4″ × 4″			L
	(plain)	Jelonet/Carbonet					
	(antibiotic)	Sofratulle		4″ × 4″			H
				4″ × 4″			H
	Cotton Wool (compressed)						
	Wound dressing (or sanitary towel)			No. 15			H
	Head dressing	Netelast		(F)			H
	Cellulose	Oxycel, Gelfoam					

	Plaster of Paris	Gypsona	emergency pack	H
	Glove (plastic)		large size	L
Cleansing				
	Soap		bar	L
Instruments				
	Scissors		blunt/sharp	M
	Forceps		oblique end	M
	Scalpel blade (sterile)		No. 15	L
	Syringes (disposable)		10 ml	L
			2 ml	L
	Needles (hypodermic)		No. 19	L
	Safety pins			L
Message				
	Pencil (wax marker)			L
	Luggage label			L

20

Emergency Messages

All written messages must be clear and succinct. A stiff luggage label or postcard and a wax crayon or very soft lead pencil should be included in all first-aid kits. They can be used in the wet and will remain readable even after rough handling.

If you reach a telephone dial 999 for the police (no money is needed) and ask for their help.

A simple message form can be devised which should carry the following information, at the minimum.

Full name and age of casualty.
Date and time of accident.
Exact location of casualty.
Map reference in 6 figures O.S.
Local geographical landmarks.
Name of climbing route.
Nature of injuries.
Treatment given.
Equipment to be brought by rescuers.
Number and condition of rest of party on the mountain.
Name of first-aider.
Map reference and telephone number where he is.

21

Safety Survival Kits

Each climber will have his own ideas about what should be carried in such a kit. Whatever the contents, the box must *live* in your rucksack and not on the shelf at home. Do not make the pack too heavy or too bulky or you will tend to avoid carrying it. Each group of items should be packed and sealed individually so that only the unit that has been broken into need be replaced. This will also discourage casual use outside the emergency situation i.e. eating the sweets or using the matches. A check list in the lid of the box will help you keep the kit complete. Each item should be labelled with simple, unambiguous instructions.

This is merely a suggested list of items; much better is to make your own.

	Individual Pack.	*Group Leader.*
		as for the Individual plus:
		Climbing rope
Shelter	Polythene bag (7′ × 3′, 120 gauge minimum)	Polythene sheet (nylon string and skewers) Bivouac tent, 'tunnel'
Direction	Map and case Compass Whistle	Flare Marker panel, fluorescent/'Dayglo' Heliograph

Message	Wax pencil and luggage label	
Light	Torch, waterproof Spare bulb and battery	Head-torch Candle, night-light
Heat	Matches, (non-safety in can with striker)	Matches, waterproof Cooker, solid fuel and spare tablets
Etc.	Penknife Tin-opener Nylon string	Wire saw Polythene water bag and plastic tube Playing cards, poker dice Needle and thread
Food	Glucose sweets (hard)	Group emergency ration Condensed milk tube
Medical	First-aid kit	First-aid kit (leader)
	In Winter:	Ice axe Crampons Goggles

Container.

A tin box can also be used as a billy-can. A screw-lid tin ensures the contents keep dry but the round tin is more difficult to pack tightly. Plastic boxes with air-tight lids are light and enable the contents to be seen.

Clothing.

Each person should also carry some spare clothing wrapped in a polythene bag to keep it dry. The minimum is a spare sweater, balaclava hat and wool socks which can double as mittens. The leader is wise to have a down jacket or sleeping bag in the bottom of his rucksack.

Index